Secret Diaries of a Nurse: and other short stories

Carolyn Ann Vaughan RN

Copyright © Carolyn Ann Vaughan RN 2015

ISBN: 978-09949443-06

To contact author:

carolyn.vaughan@ns.sympatico.ca

This book is a work of fiction the result of the authors

imagination based on life experiences.

Dedication

This book is dedicated to my family: my son

Michael, my daughters, Heather, and Melissa, my

grandsons Morgan and Devun and my soul mate and

partner David. Thank you for your support and

encouragement.

CONTENTS

THE SECRET DIARIES OF A WORKING NURSE

The Secret Diaries of a Working Nurse

By A.B.S. RN

The stories I am about to tell you are true. I have changed the names and a few of the circumstances when necessary, to protect the identity of the peoples involved. I have written this information under an assumed name. I have chosen to present this material to you in this fashion so I can be honest. This is my story.

It is also the story of many of my peers. To begin I would like to say this story is dedicated to the thousands of working nurses in Canada. Most of these nurses are women, over ninety percent of them.

Nurses are the hardest working people in Canada. A few, a very few hold cushy jobs, these are the nurses who get to call the shots, and make rules no working nurse could live with and still maintain a job.

The nurses I am talking about are the nurses who arrive at work and literally run, from task to task, yet continue to smile, even when their heart is breaking. I have nursed literally thousands of people in my thirty years as a Registered Nurse. A patient has rarely harmed me, mentally, physically, or emotionally. I am a patient advocate. I have a sore back, swollen feet, a broken heart, as well as a heart filled with joy. I am the lady with the lamp. When I die, I would like a flame placed upon my grave and an inscription that says, "she was a nurse"

I would like to describe for you the ideal nursing day. One I have yearned for but have never had the opportunity to see.

I arrived for work today, well rested. When I came on the unit, my colleagues welcomed me with a smile. They were relaxed the ward was quiet. The patients were being well cared for. The taped and written report was accurate, concise, and easily understood. Each patient wore a nametag attached to their wrists; all those with true allergies had bracelets. I'V's dripped smoothly.

I had a patient assignment of six patients. I was able to take each and every break allotted. I had time to sit with the dying, I had time to laugh with the joyful, and I had time to cry with the bereaved. In my whole day, not once did I doubt my actions. I was able to read every doctors order, because the orders were typed clearly. The Doctors rounds were conducted with ease. Each physician was polite, courteous and relaxed. There were a few crisis moments, but all the staff involved was able to handle their responsibilities with knowledge, care and precision and the patients were well served.

I sat down with my patients and actually together we developed a true plan of care, a collaborative effort with achievable goals that could be met. Every question I had about patient care was easily answered.

The CEO and my nursing supervisor congratulated me on a job well done. The housekeeping and dietary staff were friendly and supportive. The lab and the techs were relaxed and congenial, all reports were filed and ready for me. I had the opportunity to assess the patient's readiness for discharge, and I had the leisure to make certain the patients being discharged understood precisely what their discharge medications were for, and understood clearly any follow up requirements.

All ambulance and paramedics were kind, congenial and relaxed. An available and competent RN easily replaced the staff sick call for nights, and when I left the ward at the end of the day, I knew I had completed all necessary work. God, tis a glorious day. What a wonderful job nursing is! It is such a treat to be a nurse. Nursing is a job I would recommend to anyone. In your dreams Alice, in your dreams, only in your dreams does the day go like this.

Now lets tell you about the reality of today. Just today one day in the life of a Canadian nurse. I arrived, tired out, I didn't sleep well last night, I bounce from days to nights, rarely do I get a decent nights or days sleep. The ward was a zoo, we were working short staffed again.

There had been a sick call but there was no one to replace. The look of fear on the faces of my colleagues in the report room was true and genuine, the grumbling started immediately even with a full staff complement the day would be exhausting, short staffed it would be impossible.

We would survive; of course we would we had no choice. We would all have liked to pack up our purses and cell phones and leave immediately, but you can lose your license for abandonment, so of course, we could not. I said a quick and silent prayer for guidance and the help of unseen angels.

I would need it, we all would. I was charge nurse. I had only been at the institution for a month, I shouldn't be charge but I was. One patient was actively dying; three patients were in the intensive care unit, two on cardiac monitors. The long-term area was filled to capacity with mostly elderly females and most of the patients needed two workers to turn, change incontinent pads, and bathe them.

There were four people who needed to be fed, thank God one feeder was on a day pass. All the available acute beds were filled. There once was a time when an RN worked either acute, long term, ICU, CCU, or ER, but with cutbacks and juggling, todays RN in rural hospitals does it all.

We were short an IV pump because the paramedics had not yet returned the one they had borrowed for a transfer.

I smiled feebly at a student nurse she knew she would have to accept more responsibility than she was truly trained for. One RN would cover out patients and EMERG; maybe we could squeeze in a break or two, maybe.

The night nurse gave a taped report, but we couldn't hear it very well, the tape recorder was acting up, it should have been replaced or repaired, a requisition had been sent but a replacement had not yet arrived. There were little sticky notes with important information attached to each page of the Kardex.

There was one elderly lady lying on a

stretcher we didn't have a bed for her, and another was on the way from the OPD. There were a couple of PICC lines but the dressings didn't need changing today, thank God. However we had to take care of some decubitus ulcer dressings it couldn't be helped.

At least half of the acute patients had IV meds that needed to be mixed and the aerosol treatments would be time consuming. A few diabetics, but only one really counted, the one on Insulin. Some IV Lasix, some IV digoxin, and a bag that needed potassium chloride mixed to it. One error and serious complications would result.

Today would be another survival of the fittest, like the day before that, and the day before that.

Remember to smile, and be sure to give at least a few moments to the family member sitting the death watch and don't forget to thank God a family member is sitting with your dying patient.

Thank God somebody can do it, I wish I could, and I'm sorry Flo, I'm finding it harder and harder to be "loyal to my work and devoted towards the welfare of those committed to my care. "

Yours truly Alice B. Sadly RN

THE END

ALMA MAE AND THE COMPUTER

By Carolyn Ann Vaughan RN

Her arthritic fingers trembled as she read the registered letter from the tax department advising her "because of past due property taxes" her home would be put up for sale unless she paid the twelve-hundred-dollar tax bill by next Monday.

It wasn't the first letter Alma had received from the tax department. There had been others, but Alma had ignored them--all but this last one.   When she received this one, threatening a sale, she telephoned the tax department and told the young girl, who finally answered, "there must be a mistake. My husband Markus always paid his bills . . . always!"

In the fifty years they had been married, she had never once worried about bills. Markus always took care of such things.

Slowly, Alma lowered her body into the rocking chair Marcus gave her for their second wedding anniversary.

A thousand memories flooded her mind.

Where had her life gone? It seemed only yesterday the children were following Markus to the barn to feed the stock.

Alma Mae Sawler stroked the scarred wood of the old rocking chair. She'd nursed four babies in the old rocker, the twins, born in 1954, and then the boys, Andrew and William. Hot tears rolled down her wizened cheeks. Betty, the first twin died of crib death at two months of age.

Andrew and William both left the farm in the '70s. Andrew went to Sudbury to work in the nickel mines and William went to Northern B.C. to work for Alcan.

Her eldest twin daughter Jean had stayed in Nova Scotia, gone to teacher's college, and taught at St. Patrick's high school in Halifax.

She'd taught for twenty years until she died of breast cancer almost three years ago.

Carefully, Alma folded the letter and placed it in the pocket of her calico apron-the apron Jean gave her one-year for Mother's Day. The cloth was worn soft and the colours faded, but it was Alma's favourite. She wore it often.

Alma covered her face with her hands and let the tears flow, so many memories, and so many losses. Markus gone now, she'd buried him in the family plot just this past winter, beside infant Betty and Jean.

The boys had come home for their father's funeral. They had stayed on the farm with her for more than a week; it was all the time they could get off from their work.

The boys had taken turns trying to get her to move, but she had refused. Andrew's wife, Caroline, had even hinted that Alma was being selfish by not agreeing to move in with them.

Alma snuffled a soft keening sound. She'd never liked Andrew's wife very much. Of course it wasn't Caroline's fault really; Caroline just wasn't a Maritimer.

No, Alma Mae was not going to leave Nova Scotia. She wouldn't know how to live anywhere else. Seven generations of her family had worked and toiled on the land and on the sea. She was of Planter stock with roots going back even before the empire loyalists. She was born in Nova Scotia; she would die in Nova Scotia.

William, too, had tried to persuade her to move, but she knew she would miss the sea. William told her there was a great big ocean in Northern B.C. but still Alma refused.

The Pacific wasn't her ocean. Alma Mae knew every rock on her small piece of Atlantic coastline. She knew her land, where the blueberries grew, and where the old barn had stood. She knew where they had buried the last farm horse. And every year for almost fifty years she watched snowfalls bend the boughs of the old pine tree that hovered beyond the wild roses. And every year she filled the bird feeder for the blue jays that came to feed. No, she wouldn't move from her home. Never!

She didn't use the upstairs portion of the

house anymore. She and Markus had moved their bedroom downstairs two winters ago, after he suffered his first heart attack.

Sometimes on a clear day, when her arthritic knees would allow it, she would climb the stairs and gaze out across the water to the point of land where her grandfather once told her he always placed his lobster pots. No one would move her from her home . . . no one!

Alma dried her tears with the edge of her apron. She could call William, or even Andrew; they would know what to do. They would fix the tax letter. Yes, that's what she would do; she would call William in B.C. She wouldn't call Andrew; she didn't want to talk to Caroline, didn't want to give that girl more fuel than necessary.

She would fix herself a cup of chamomile tea, and then she would make her telephone call. But first, before she called, she would try using the computer. Markus had shown her how to send email. She didn't like the computer; it wasn't the same as talking to William. Still, maybe the computer would be easier than talking to him.

Carefully she carried her tea and a piece of homemade bread with crab apple jelly to the office nook. How many times had she carried a simple meal to Markus in this very same spot as he worked on the accounts?

As if it were yesterday, she remembered the pride on his face as he put up the shelves to hold the books about animal husbandry. If she closed her eyes she could see the first big, old black telephone and she recalled if the phone rang three times it was for them. If the black box phone rang two long and one short ring it was for Annabelle Parsons.

A smile crossed her face remembering how Jean always complained that; Annabelle listened in on her telephone calls. Alma doubted Annabelle ever listened to a young girl's secrets, but Jean was sure she did. Even Annabelle was gone now: she moved to Toronto to be with her grandchildren when her own husband died.

Alma Mae put the cup down on the weathered desktop. With the tip of her finger, she traced the crude heart shape William had carved in the pine when he was just a little boy. There was a smell of old wood and old books in the little nook. But there were also the blinking lights of a brand new computer.

Well, maybe not new. Markus had purchased it three years ago. He said it made the bookwork so much easier. Dear, sweet Markus, a man with big hands, fisherman's hands, and a face weathered by wind and rain. Even in old age his eyes were the blue of forget me not flowers.

The tax people were wrong! They had to be! Alma knew her husband. Never in all the years they had lived together, never had he ever failed to pay a bill. Sometimes he was late, that was the nature of farming and fishing. But he always paid. Always!

The young snippet in the tax department had told her the computer did not lie, and her property taxes were not paid. But Alma knew. She knew that somehow, in some way the computer had lied this time. It had to, because her Markus never lied. Of that truth, Alma Mae was certain.

Gingerly she reached for the slim book that held the accounts. Markus started a new book every five years. Every penny the family had ever received, and every expense ever paid, was listed. There it was, written in his own hand writing, "$1,237.00, three years property tax paid in full Aug. 3, - online."

Alma studied the writing. Markus had paid the bill, it was written in his account book just three days before he died. Alma had told the girl at the tax office Markus had paid it, but the snippet had said maybe he was about to pay it and had written it in ahead of time. But Alma knew Markus. He wouldn't do that. If Markus had written, "Paid in full," it <u>was</u> paid in full.

Alma Mae scanned the records. Some of the entries were listed as "paid online." Power, telephone, the heat bill, each of these stated "paid online." Alma could feel the tremble of her heart, and her mouth got dry.

She remembered the glee in his eye when he talked about the marvel of on-line banking. He loved technology, her Markus did. He said it was the future. He had shown her once how to access their on-line bank account. Alma had preferred to walk in to the bank and speak to a teller; but still Markus had insisted. He had even written precise instructions for exactly how to open the online account, and see the balance.

Alma Mae made her choice--she would use the machine. Gingerly, she turned it on. The pages flashed before her eyes. There was a little picture for banking; she flicked the button as Markus had shown her. The screen came up asking for a password.

She turned to the first page of the account book and there in his hand was the password. The file showed the two accounts, a savings account, $437.53, and the chequing account holding $123.32. Alma was delighted; she knew that was the exact amount she had in the bank.

She studied the screen; she knew there had to be more. He had told her distinctly he had paid bills online. Then she saw it off to the left, under bills. She tapped the button and a list of creditors flashed on the screen, Maritime Tel and Tel, Nova Scotia Power, Sears, Cummings Insurance. Finally she saw it, Municipal Taxes and . . . a message, one that caused her to spill a little of her tea on the apron Jean had given her. Before her eyes, beside the property taxes, in small print, were the words, "wrong merchant." Alma could almost hear Markus whisper in her ear, "You've got it, Alma Mae, you've got it." And Alma was just about positive she had found the mistake.

There had to be a way to print this, she had seen Marcus do it more than once. She studied the printer, pressed the "on" button, and located the onscreen print button. In moments a page was printed showing the creditors, but most importantly showing the message "wrong merchant" beside the Municipal taxes.

Alma breathed a sigh of relief: her home, her precious home was not in the Municipality--it was in the County. Somehow, in some way, a mistake had been made and she, Alma Mae Sawler, would get to the bottom of it.

Alma set her teacup in the sink, donned her best dress, and picked up her pocket book . . . and her precious printout. The drive to the bank was filled with thoughts of Markus.

When she arrived, the bank was short on customers and she marched straight up to the teller and demanded to see the bank manager, Clyde Barkhouse.

"Yes, Alma," he said, brushing a fleck of dust from his pin-stripped tie. "What can we do for you this morning?"

Alma shoved the paper closer. "This is the record of the back taxes Markus paid. If I understand it correctly, there has been an error."

Clyde sighed deeply, "It would be quite unlikely Alma. You know here at the bank we use computers and of course the technology is incredibly accurate and does not make mistakes."

Alma shoved her paper a tiny bit closer.

"I know you use computers Clyde. But, Clyde, the computer has lied. Now, I suggest you look at this record . . . because my Markus does not lie."

Clyde picked up the papers and Alma watched his face. She could see by the twitch of an eyebrow, he had seen the mistake.

"Hmm . . . It would appear there may have been a slight problem. I'll have to make a few phone calls."

"I suggest you do that, and I'll wait over here," Alma said, gesturing to a couple of orange plastic chairs beneath the plate glass window. The bank manager disappeared into his office. Alma sat in the chair reading an old copy of Canadian Gardening magazine.

Half-hour later, a red-faced Clyde approached her. "It seems your records are correct," he said. "The money was deducted from your account and the funds were sent to the municipal tax department instead of the County.

The municipality has been holding the funds and will forward them immediately to the appropriate tax office. Do you wish to file an official complaint?"

Alma rose from her chair, considering the question. "No, Clyde, I do not. But," she added, "a letter of apology stating that the computer

And not my Markus 'lied,' would be in order."

And with that Alma Mae Sawler turned and marched out the door into the summer sunshine of her North Atlantic Coast.

The End

CONVERSATIONS

WITH GERALD

Taking Stock In January

By Carolyn Ann Vaughan RN

I dropped in to visit with my friend Gerald; he was seated at his kitchen table, a notebook open in front of him. "What are you doing today Gerald?" I asked, as he poured me a cup of tea.

"Taking stock of things to rejoice about."

I smiled and asked, "taking stock of what Gerald?"

"All the good things I see in life."

I sipped the freshly brewed tea and waited. "Sometimes Gerald," I said, "It seems hard to see the good things. Every time I open a paper or watch the news I see sorrow, anger, fear, all sorts of things, much that doesn't seem worthy of rejoicing."

"Yes," he said scratching his bearded stubble, "this sometimes seems true."

"But," he said with a twinkle in his watery blue eyes, "do you also see the beauty, the joy and the wonder of things?"

He walked over to his kitchen sink and turned on the water, and for a moment he let the water run over his hand. "You see this water Carolyn, "I once had a house guest who told me in the

African village where he was raised his mother had to walk almost half a day to get clean water for her family."

He shuffled to his cupboard, opened it and pointed to the canned goods stacked on the shelf. "See these food items here, I recall a young refuge once telling me she and her family were so hungry when they fled their country they had to eat field mice to survive."

He placed a few sweetbreads on a plate, opened his refrigerator and selected a jar of homemade jam. Placing it before me, he said. "This here jam was made by me granddaughter Lindsay. She picked the berries herself and made what she called freezer jam." He gave me a little grin, "I remember the day the wife and I got our first refrigerator, it was an exciting moment. What a luxury a refrigerator was he said, shaking his head, what a luxury."

We ate our simple meal of tea and sweetbreads and Gerald once again rose from his seat and walked over to the thermostat.

"I'm not saying we don't have issues to deal with in this country Carolyn, we do. Lots of em I suppose, health care, the environment, crime, worthwhile jobs."

"But," he said, touching the thermostat; "see how easy I can make this home a little warmer. Do you know my granddaddy had to work all year to harvest, season, and chop wood just to keep his family warm in the winter?" He smiled once again, "I just turn this little dial and out comes the heat. Isn't that a wonder?"

For just a moment, I could picture Gerald's granddaddy chopping wood and marveled at the wonder of turning a dial to warm a room. Gerald returned to his seat and pushed yesterday's newspaper towards me.

The headlines blared about the upcoming election.

"And this," he said, pointing to the headlines, "this gets added to all the other things I take stock of this January."

"An election, how could an election be something to take stock of or rejoice about? Most folks are grumbling about a winter election and heaven knows there's an awful lot of negative talk, one political group blasting another about the failures."

"Yep he said, tis true, but think about it Carolyn, do you know in some parts of this world people have fought wars just to be able to vote. Why even in this country I remember my grandmother telling of the efforts the ladies went through just to be allowed to vote. Now that my girl, that is something. Do you know today a woman can cast a vote, why she can even choose to run for elected office? My grandmother would have called that a miracle."

I finished the last of my tea and placed the cup and saucer in the sink.

"You come on back election night," he said, "the wife and I will make us a wee snack. We'll settle in front of the coloured television set and right before our very eyes, we'll be able to watch the election. Think about it, Carolyn right here in my very own home I can watch the Canadian people chose. That," he said, "is also something worth taking stock of this January."

GERALD AND CAR INSURANCE

By Carolyn Ann Vaughan RN

The other day I bought a three thousand dollar car to get myself back and forth to work. The insurance company told me it would cost $838.00 a year to insure it. I was feeling dismayed, thinking the cost of the insurance was almost a third of the price of the transportation, when I saw my neighbour Gerald out in his yard loading brush into the back of his pick up.

Gerald I said, "you have a truck in fairly good shape, what do you pay for insurance?

Gerald took a swipe at his whiskery chin and said, "Well, used to pay twelve hundred dollars a year," then he looked abashed, "didn't pay anything this year though."

"You didn't pay anything?"

"Nope, couldn't afford it. The oil company wouldn't deliver fuel last winter unless I replaced the old tank, and the missus needed some expensive medicines, so... I let the car insurance lapse."

I was shaken by what he'd said. "Gerald, doesn't it worry you to be driving without insurance?"

"Yep sure does, but you can't make blood from a turnip, and besides Carolyn, sometimes there are not many alternatives."

Gerald, I heard the Nova Scotia motor vehicle branch won't renew your registration unless you show proof of insurance, what will you do then."

"Don't right know Carolyn, rub a little mud on the sticker, get the missus to pray I don't get stopped or have an accident and hope a little more work comes my way I guess."

"And if it doesn't?"

"Worry a mite, feel angry when I read about fancy government bookkeeping, or hear there'll be another hike in gasoline prices. Go home and hug the missus, and be grateful at sixty-three I still have my health." He removed a well-used harmonica out of his red-checkered flannel shirt pocket and began to play an upbeat melody. And before long, I began to tap my toe to the music.

The sun was warm on my face, the air was clean and clear and off to the left I could hear a sparrow answer his harmonica. The music brought a smile to my lips.

"It's a tune I play when a car load of us drive to the valley during picking season. Or get a bit of woods work. It keeps our spirits up."

"Sometimes Carolyn," he said, "in this life you got to make hard choices. I wish it were not so, but I don't make the rules, I just do the best I can to live with them."

I'm grateful for my neighbour Gerald, he doesn't always have answers for me, but he helps me to put many things in perspective.

GERALD IS

RIGHT

By Carolyn Ann Vaughan RN

Gerald is Right, I just don't understand politics, therefore I try to learn from my friend Gerald, once a fisherman, now a political guru. During our chit chat the subject of legalized gambling came up. I said, "Gerald, I've heard there's a political debate going on about VLT's and Casino's."

Gerald replied. "Yep, it's kind of complicated though. It's tied up with federal inquiries, land claims and federal and provincial governments saving and spending tax money to fight organized crime."

"Oh really," I said.

"Yep, the province saved a 100 million tax dollars by not dumping the Halifax Casino. But," he added, "The folks running the Province say there's a gambling problem in Nova Scotia. So to fix it, they plan to axe a few VLT's and toss out a few more million tax dollars. You know, health promotion, maybe even have a plebiscite. Of course," he said, "the province can't do much about VLT's or casino's on reservations, unless they buy out reservation VLT's or discuss land claims, which is kinda tied up with federal issues."

I, wanting to believe in the power of governments said, "but Gerald if legalized gambling causes problems for people, can't councils and governments stop it if they want to?"

Gerald, much wiser than I in the workings of the political world said, "You know governments have to generate revenue, create jobs, support the tourist industry, provide for the welfare of their members."

I said, "Gerald, I've heard legalized gambling is creating bankruptcies, suicides, increasing drug use, all manner of social ills."

He squinted up his eyes and said, "um, well,

yep, I suppose, but well, governments, have to make trade offs you know, generate revenue."

"But Gerald," I said, "doesn't this revenue generation cause lots of problems for little people, the folks who don't make the rules. Sometimes," I said, "the whole legalized gambling issue looks pretty dirty."

Gerald scratched his chin, "that's why the good Prime Minister and the gang don't want to eradicate all legalized gambling, and there's the worry of organized crime and all those grey machines."

I said, "but Gerald, I thought historically organized crime used gambling to launder drug money."

Gerald looked contemplative and said. "Well,

organized crimes don't run gambling anymore." And he winked, then looked me in the eye and said, "little folks just need backbone, take some personal responsibility when it comes to gambling and who knows maybe government can provide some gambling resources, maybe even IT jobs to outsource, take it all offshore."

"Oh," I said. "It really is complicated, let me see if I can understand. "We once didn't have legalized gambling in Canada. Then we did have legalized gambling. Organized crimes use to run gambling, now they don't. The province thinks there's a problem and wants to help so they save some tax money and then spend some tax money.

The Feds spend our money on a big enquiry about organized crime connections and politics, but of course in Canada we don't really have organized crime.

Legalized gambling in Nova Scotia may be increasing rates of suicide, depression, drug use, bankruptcy, but it provides jobs, supports the tourist industry, could even spur IT jobs, and legalized gambling generates massive revenues, all of which benefits everyone except those who are depressed, bankrupt, become involved in the drug trade or have committed suicide," and I said, "councils and government get to keep all this generated revenue from VLT's and Casino's. Right?"

"No," he said, "it's not quite like that, the

province and the reservations only get a little of the take, they all make trade offs."

I said, "but Gerald, who gets the rest of the take."

He chewed a plug of tobacco, swallowed a thimble of homemade moonshine, pointed his finger and said, "Carolyn, your problem is, you just don't understand the concept of trade offs and politics."

I guess Gerald is right, I just don't understand politics and tradeoffs.

GERALD

NEGOTIATING

By Carolyn Ann Vaughan RN

I was sitting down having a cup of tea with my neighbour Gerald when the subject of credit cards came up.

"Gerald, what do you think of credit cards?"

"Durn nuisance," he said", Folks always spending what they don't have today and then being stuck to the proverbial grinding stone to pay it off tomorrow. Some folks even have two and three o' those plastic things and keep juggling back and forth just to keep their heads above water."

I swallowed a mouthful of my tea and said, "it does get tricky though Gerald. Just today, I received another advertisement in the mail offering me a super deal on interest rates. Seems to me it might be wise to get a different card than the one I currently have. The advertised rate is almost six percent less than what I'm paying now. What do you think?"

"Well let's see," he said, as he bit a chew of his tobacco, "you say you want to get another card cause the interest rate is lower. Have you been making regular payments on the one you gut?"

"Sure, I keep it up pretty well; you know I had

a spot of trouble with credit cards awhile back, when I was a little younger, so I try to protect my credit rating now."

"Smart girl. Best to pay cash when you can. And keep the card in your pocket for emergencies, things like false teeth and such. But I knows in this day and age it's thorny to live without the durn things. But," he said, "you don't have to take the rate they offer you; all you gotta do is make one phone call. Try a little negotiating."

"Make one phone call?"

"Sure. Call em; tell em you're not happy with your current interest rate. And ask em if there's any reason why you shouldn't switch to a company that offers a lower rate."

"Surely, that wouldn't work."

"Worked for me."

"Honestly?"

"Yep, I called em on their toll free number, asked em why I shouldn't switch to a card with a lower rate. They hemmed and hawed for a few minutes, and then dropped my interest rate by six percent, even told me they'd make it retroactive to my last statement. Said I was a good customer and they wanted to keep my business. 'Fore you go getting another card just cause of the lower interest rate, Carolyn, try a little negotiating."

After Gerald left and I washed up our teacups, I did just as he suggested, and called the Credit card Company. I asked if I had the best interest rate they could offer and mentioned I was contemplating taking advantage of some of the credit card deals that kept arriving in the mail.

The credit card company employee did just as Gerald said they would. They hemmed and hawed a little, passed me on to another employee and then dropped my monthly interest rate by five percent.

I was delighted. I plan to use the interest I saved this month to buy my friend Gerald a forsythia plant for his flower garden. Sometimes, Gerald is right; when it comes to credit cards it makes sense to do a little negotiating.

GERALD ON

WORK

By Carolyn Ann Vaughan RN

"Gerald," I said, "you've had a lot of different jobs. What do you think is the toughest job you've ever had?"

Gerald contemplated the tip of his battered work boots, got a far a way look in his eye and took a long time answering.

"Well," he said, "let's see, I cut ice for awhile back in the day when they needed big blocks for Ice chests. If I recollect rightly we cut the blocks from the Dartmouth Lakes. That was cold work."

He pulled a plug of Redman chewing tobacco out of his plaid jacket and said. "Then I had a chance to work for a year or so helping build the old Angus L. Bridge, round about the middle fifties, course that job came to an end when they got the bridge finished up."

"Yep," he said, "remember trying my hand at selling gidgets and gadgets door to door, but never quite got the hang of it, least not enough to support the family." He studied his calloused hands, "worked in the mines for a bit, that was rugged work, good pay, but couldn't do it for long though." He looked away, as if remembering an embarrassment.

"And," he said, "I spent a few seasons in the logging camps. Food was good, cook always saw to that but I was away from home for weeks at a time. The missus didn't like that much. We had seven children, three girls and four boys. So then I drove a snowplow for a few winters and did farm labour, mostly during apple season."

He stood a little taller, "me back was a tad better in those days" he said with a grin. "Aw yes, helped old Jake Gillis with shingling roofs for awhile twas hard on the knees. Oh yes almost forgot about driving a fuel delivery truck, had to watch out for dogs, people didn't always tie em up. Yes I spect I've had a few different jobs in my day. Guess I pretty much did whatever I put my hand to".

He caressed the stub of his index finger, "did some mill work for awhile, till I got in a fight with the power saw, lost the tip of my finger in that row, and of course I worked on the fishin' boats back when fish was plentiful." He stopped to take plug fro his Red Man pouch.

"Yep, lots of work, this and that. The missus and I did whatever we could to keep a roof over our heads and food in the belly."

Gerald reached over and gave my hand a pat. "You know Carolyn, I've done lots of jobs, but when I really think about it, the hardest job I ever had was raisin, the young uns."

"Somehow, the missus and I managed to raise em all. Didn't lose a one of em, came close when Samuel got in trouble with the law, and Rebecca started her family fore she was a mind too.

Worried a lot the missus and I, when young Henry left for Sudbury to work in the nickel mines and Mary Beth got hooked up with the fella who liked his moonshine but you know, the truth is, the hardest job I ever had was doing me best for the family."

"You know," he said, a look of awe on his face, "there'll be twenty two of em here for Father's Day dinner, that me girl," he said, "being a father and a family man sometimes, that was

me hardest job."

GERALD'S

LETTERS

By Carolyn Ann Vaughan RN

I stopped at the end of Gerald's driveway, picked up his mail handed it to him anticipating a neighbourly chat with my elderly friend.

"Well, I'll be," he said, "It seems I got me a couple of letters from away, one from old Sam MacDonald. He writes me every now an again, and the other from my Grandson, Jeremy."

"You have that nostalgic look in your eye Gerald; I know I feel a story coming on."

Gerald tugged at his whiskers, "um, I suppose there is a story. You see Sam and I come from a generation when going down the road meant going to the New England states."

"You mean folks once left Nova Scotia for New England? I always thought going down the road meant heading for Ontario."

"Nah, that was your generation, Carolyn. My generation went to the New England states, Maine, New Jersey, Boston mostly, and of course me grandkids go to the streets paved in Gold way out in Alberta"

Gerald gave his red suspenders a flick, "I almost went with old Sam MacDonald to the

U.S. of A, I was a young pup then, not much work around these parts, and I spect I was looking for a bit of excitement.

"What stopped you?"

Gerald, chewed on his lip, "suppose it was because I was sweet on the missus, course she wasn't the missus then," he said with a grin.

"Sam MacDonald ended up in Boston, he's a Yankee now I guess, been there since 1942, course he comes home once in awhile but he made a life for himself in the United States. Course back in 1942, Canada was quite different from the United States." Gerald sipped, his tea, "not so sure that's really the case today."

"Did he ever regret his move Gerald?"

"Yep, it was in the fall of 1971, he lost his son to Vietnam, he never wanted his son to go to war, but the Americans had a different system back then, not like today. Soldiering is voluntary now, well sort of I suppose, fella's still gotta have a job I spect so they still sometimes go where the work is."

"Yes Gerald, it seems maritimers are always hungry for work. I know my brother took a spin at Ontario, but it didn't last long, he got awful tired of the dirt and grind of shift work at the auto plant, he came back home after a few years, he always says he misses the money though."

"Yep, a job with good paying money seems to cause a lot of wandering for us Nova Scotians.

My grandson Jeremy is out in Alberta says there are all kinds of jobs out there, but his wife is homesick for the Maritimes. She was okay until the babies came along, now she feels kind of at sea without a sail, so he says."

"Do you think there is ever going to be any solution to Maritime wanderings Gerald?"

Gerald took out a plug of chewing tobacco and said, "I heard the other day someone thought the government should pay travel expenses for those unemployed who want to find work out west. Then there's another group of business folks talking about something they call Atlantica. I guess that's some kind of different trade with the New England states, supposed to make the Maritimes a little more prosperous, so they think."

"Do you believe either of those ideas have merit Gerald?"

"Well, now, you know I can't rightly say. People have a need for decent work that's for sure. For lots of reasons, shelter, food, structure and a sense of self-esteem and accomplishment, but to my way of looking at it, they also need family and a life style and identity they feel they can live with. Guess I'll just have to watch, wait and see. But I'm somewhat relieved my own job hunting days are over though."

"Some tea Carolyn?"

LIGHTENING

THE LOAD

By Carolyn Ann Vaughan RN

"Heh, Gerald, what are you doing?"

"Well Carolyn, I am lightening the load."

"But Gerald, you're just hanging your tools on a peg board. I can see how that might help a little but why do you say you're lightening the load?"

Gerald scratched his whiskers and gave a snap to his red suspenders. "Sometimes when you get a little older Carolyn you learn a trick or two about how to keep daily frustrations at a minimum."

"What kind of tricks, Gerald?"

"Well let's see now, tricks like having a peg board to hang me tools on, that way I don't have to go all over searching for em when I need em," he said with a grin. "Stuff like making sure I have a nail to hang my truck keys on, cleaning off my garden tools at the end of the season, emptying the gas from my mower, writing down the garbage pick up day on my calendar."

"Doesn't all that attention to small detail take

time?"

"Yep, you bet, but it saves a lot of frustration time too. For instance, I know where my tools and my keys are when I need em and my garden equipment is ready for next year. I call it lightening me load. Took me quite a few years to put into practice some of the tricks though.

"Gerald are you saying organization in small things make the bigger challenges easier to handle?

"Yep, guess that's what I'm saying. You see there once was a time when I didn't spend a few minutes thinking ahead and my life became chaotic. I could never find a clean shirt. I spent a lot of time searching for my truck keys, or my hip waders and half the time I ran out of milk and eggs. Then I'd be in a sour mood for the rest of the day all because I didn't practice lightening the load. And of course, when a big problem came along I was totally swamped."

"I don't know Gerald, sometimes it seems like life is a matter of dashing from one issue to another. I don't see how I could ever get organized."

"You don't have to do everything at once Carolyn, just one little trick at a time, when you get that un down pat, you take on another. I'll give you the little tip I told the missus the other day, maybe it will work for you. When I do the laundry, I always put the shirts on plastic hangers before putting em on the clothesline, or taking em out of the dryer that way they just go straight to the closet. It saves folding em, never did like trying to fold shirts much.

"Heh thanks Gerald; I think I'll try that, who knows maybe if I get better control of the little things the big issues won't be so overwhelming."

"Works for me Carolyn, that's why I call it lightening me load."

MY SHIP HAS

COME IN

By Carolyn Ann Vaughan RN

"Gerald, Gerald," I shouted, barging into his kitchen. "Look, I've just won 7 million British pounds!" I was so excited I could barely contain myself. "See," I said shoving the paper into his arthritic hands. "See, it says right here, 7 million British pounds. I'm, loaded, Gerald, just plain loaded. My ship has finally come in."

"Whoa, slow down lass, have a seat and let's ponder this thing just a little."

"But Gerald," I exclaimed, "The email note says I <u>definitely won.</u> It doesn't say maybe, or I have a chance or anything like that. It says right here in black and white. Your email address has been chosen as a winner." I was so excited I could hardly keep from jumping up and down.

"All I have to do," I said, "is call this overseas telephone number on this sheet of paper to confirm my winnings and they will send me the money."

"Um, he said, as he flicked his red suspenders," did you buy a ticket or enter any contests lately."

"Well ...No" I admitted, "but look, right here it says they selected my email from a random draw of thousands of online organizations."

"Um," his watery blue eyes crinkled at the corners.

"I belong to a number of organizations that have online sites Gerald, and besides" I added, "the National Lottery is a genuine British Lottery, sort of like our Atlantic lotto."

"You don't seem very excited Gerald?"

He took a plug of chewing tobacco from his

green plaid work shirt and replied. "Not to rain on your parade or anything missy, but I think we need to verify this here note, before you go making long distance telephone calls or booking cruises to the sunny south."

"I suppose your right." I said grudgingly, "but I'm pretty sure it's on the up and up. I mean the letter looks so completely sincere. Fantastical and wonderful I admit, but sincere."

He smiled, poured me a cup of tea and glancing at the paper I handed him, he said, "Yup, it sure is one smooth talking letter."

Taking the letter and shuffling towards his rolled top desk, Gerald sat down at his computer and in a moment, he had pulled up the web site of the British national lottery. The address was the same as on my email notification.

"See, Gerald," I said. "It is a real place!"

Then with the flick of a mouse, he hit the box labeled scams. And before my very eyes, almost word for word, listed under Internet scams, I read my letter.

"Oh, Gerald," I wailed, "My letter is an out and out scam. I was certain my ship finally arrived at home port."

"Seems to me, he said, "I'd say you saved yourself the cost of a long distance phone call, maybe a courier's bill and who knows what other manner of troubles."

Then he flashed me a crooked grin, scratched his grizzly white whiskers and said, "Yup, Carolyn, seems to me he said, "Your ship managed to avoid going aground on a sand bar."

"Guess when all's said and done," he said, "your ship will survive to sail another day."

"More tea Missy"

THE WAY THINGS ARE DONE NOWADAYS

By Carolyn Ann Vaughan RN

"What are you doing Gerald, you seem unusually troubled today?"

"Yes, Lass, I admit I am. I'm writing a letter to my cousin Alma to try and cheer her up."

"Why does Alma need Cheering?"

"Well Lass, she has a problem, a big one by the looks of it. You see she and her husband Joe have been sent to different nursing homes. One is in Bridgewater the other is in Truro."

"How did that come about Gerald?"

"Oh, lass it's the way things are done nowadays."

"What do you mean, they way things are done. Didn't they want to be together?"

"Yep, they sure did, but there was a glitch in the way their case was handled and now one is a resident in a nursing home in Truro and the other is a resident in Bridgewater. Joe needs a little more care than Alma and there just weren't any openings in a facility where they could both be together."

"Isn't there anything that can be done Gerald?"

"Well," he said, scratching his whiskery chin, "all the official type folks keep promising them they are working on it. But it is getting to be pretty hard on Alma. She's 82 this spring and she and Joe have not been separated before. It has been almost six weeks and it seems like a mighty long stretch. I understand she cries a lot and asks all the nurses and doctors when the situation will change."

"How do they manage Gerald?"

"They talk on the phone everyday, sometimes two or three times a day, but Joe isn't as strong mentally as he once was. I worry about them, what with the weather getting warmer and all."

"What do you mean the weather getting warmer?"

"Well lass I fear Alma may take it upon herself to try and leave the home, and somehow make her way to Bridgewater. Joe wouldn't be able to get away; he's in one of those special wards where the doors are locked. He has a tendency to wander at times, but well, Alma she is able to come and go a little more and I just don't think is able to be patient enough to wait for the process that will allow them to be together."

"Gerald, I just don't see how this could possibly happen. Don't the powers that be understand the situation?"

"Oh sure lass, they understand but nursing

home beds are difficult to come by, often there is a waiting list and sometimes people have to take the first bed that comes along."

"This means people who have spent all their lives in a particular community might have to accept a bed in another community."

"Isn't this difficult for elderly people?"

"Yep, it sure is, and it means a lot of shuffling back and forth for old folks. But apparently, it saves money for the health care system."

"How does it save money Gerald?

"Well, the financial costs of keeping folks in a hospital bed is more expensive than keeping folks in a nursing home bed so if a couple is in a hospital but they really need a nursing home they are required to take the first available bed and in Joe and Alma's case they ended up in different communities separated by hundred of miles."

"Oh Lord, Gerald that sounds so, well, I guess heartless is the word I am thinking of."

"Yes, lass, I suppose it tis, but that's the way the system works nowadays."

Then he licked the stamp and placed it on his letter. "I just hope they can wait it out eventually they will be together again. But Joe can't understand the way he once could so a day separated from Alma seems like a lifetime and," he said his blue eyes troubled, "it breaks my heart to hear the angst in their voices when I speak to them."

"They're good people, Joe and Alma, paid their taxes, and raised their children, contributed to the community. It's not the way it should be done Carolyn. No, tis not but perhaps next week, they will get the news that they can be together again. It is my hope; if not, maybe, I'll try contacting the minister of health. In the meantime we wait and we hope and we pray."

A STUMPER FOR

GERALD

By Carolyn Ann Vaughan R.N.

"Gerald, I have a stumper for you. What do you think is the greatest marketing tool of all time?"

Gerald paused a moment, snapped his red suspenders and said. "Eh lass, that's an easy one. The greatest marketing tool of all time is fear."

"Uh," I said with raised eyebrow. "Fear?"

"Sure, think about it, everything sold, from warships, to insurance, to low fat foods, to pharmaceuticals works because someone is selling fear."

"Wow, Gerald, I don't know about your answer. I think I might have chosen greed or even plain old desire as a sales pitch."

"Na, greed or desire might play a tiny part, but to really grab a customer by the shirt tail you have to appeal to their fears."

"Well what about the phenomenal sales of the pet rock, or a toy surely those sales aren't motivated by fear."

"Oh sure they are," he said with a puff of his whiskered cheeks, "the fear of missing out on something unique, or the fear of letting your child down."

Gerald took a bite of his Red Man chewing tobacco and after contemplating for a while he said. "You know, come to think of it, maybe even the sales pitch of a politician or a preacher works best when it dishes up a little fear."

"Oh come now Gerald my friend, surely you're kidding me!"

He chewed for a while and then said, "Nope." Not kidding, it's our own fears that trap us. Instilling fear is sure to catch us every time. Causes all manner of problems and sure to be profitable when someone can find a way to market it."

"Well, Gerald," I said, "If your theory is correct is their anything a person can do about fear?"

"Yep, but it ain't easy, I been working on it for neigh on seventy years and still ain't conquered it yet."

"What do you do?"

"Well, I try to live one day at a time, helps quite a bit." Then he said, " I attend to the small things. That way stuff doesn't pile up too much. And of course I make an effort to live simply. Oh yeah, and I be sure to make amends with folks before the sun goes down."

He poured himself a cup of his famous tea and said, "I take responsibility for the tough choices I sometimes have to make and I be sure my choices allow me to face myself in the mirror at the end of the day."

"How does that help with fear?" I asked.

"It allows me not to fear me conscience, course it means sometimes I have to forgive me self for human frailty." And he said, "One of my biggest fear busters is to rejoice in diversity, respecting differences of choice or opinion among all manner of folk."

Gerald sipped a little of the tea that had fallen into his saucer and continued, "By lending a hand, or a prayer or the coat in me closet I keep busy enough to avoid a lot of the sales pitches."

And he added. "Perhaps my best tool is to trust me instincts and look for that of good in all peoples" then he said with a crooked grin, "sometimes when I get terribly overloaded with the sales pitches selling fear, I need to spend a little time alone, with just the birds, the stars and me harmonica. That usually puts things in perspective."

GERALD AND ASSETS

By Carolyn Ann Vaughan RN

The other day, while Gerald and I were sitting down to a cup of tea, I showed him a book I had been reading about financial security.

"Gerald," I said, "my book suggests a person make a periodic check of their assets and keep a list. I was wondering if you've ever spent any time tallying your assets."

"Oh sure," he said, "I have a list of my assets hanging right there over by the telephone."

"Gerald," I said, "that's a telephone list of your friends and neighbours."

"Yep"

"But Gerald, I think the book is referring to things like money in the bank, a home, a car, maybe some RRSP's or stock options, perhaps an insurance policy, something with cash value."

"Well," he said, scratching his chin, "I suppose that is one kind of asset but don't seem to me to be the sort of stuff with much real value."

Then he asked, "Does your book say anything

about people being an asset?"

"No, Gerald, people aren't listed as assets because, well.... because they don't have cash value."

"Um, maybe they don't have cash value but a few good friends and a supportive family are worth more than all the tea in china and I'd druther have these than a fine home, or a big bank roll."

"So Gerald are you are telling me you consider friends and family more valuable than a house or a car or stock options."

"Yep, guess that's what I'm telling you. You see Carolyn, people can offer advice, baby-sit the children if need be, bring you a little home made soup when you're under the weather.

Maybe help when the car gets stuck in the snow."

He added. "Folks can offer you a shoulder to lean on when life gets tough, or trade a work shift, seems to me it really isn't any contest. People and relationships count as far more valuable than stock options or big homes."

"So Gerald, are you saying people are more valuable than a bank account."

"Yep, guess that's what I'm saying. Don't get me wrong, it's nice to have a nest egg, but the way I see it, true security comes in the comforting words and help of people when the going gets tough."

Then with a grin he said, "Course your book might not see it like this and I suppose your book would advise you to put all your efforts into attaining the things they call assets, but it don't convince me much."

He hitched up his red suspenders and said, "I've lived long enough to know it's more important to have a neighbour who will help me get the tractor out of the ditch. Or visit the missus when she gets a little lonely. So sure Carolyn, I keep a list of me assets, I make sure it hangs right there by my telephone."

"Yep," he said, "that's me assets, and I update my list every couple of years or so, would you like a little more tea Carolyn?"

GERALD'S

CHRISTMAS

By Carolyn Ann Vaughan RN

I had spent a hectic day battling crowds at the mall, wondering if I had done all the things, I felt needed to be done to have a wonderful holiday. I was tired and just a little cranky and on my way home, I stopped off to visit my neighbour Gerald. His kitchen was warm and inviting with nary a Christmas decoration in sight but he was pouring a small amount of liquid over a dark fruitcake. "Gerald," I asked "don't you celebrate the Holidays?"

"Oh sure," he said, "but I guess the missus and I celebrate a little different from other folks."

"What do you mean?"

Gerald added a stick of firewood to the kitchen range and said with a grin "for starters we always make our own fruit cake," he said, pouring a little rum over the top of the cake. "This here cake will have a nice mellow flavor when you let it sit a few weeks." Then he wrapped the cake in cheesecloth and returned it to an airtight container.

"In the old days they use to call it war cake,

the women folk would make the cakes and send them overseas to the men at the front. I remember a cake just like this un that my ma made back in the Christmas of 42."

"What else do you do at Christmas Gerald?"

"Well we make our own candy, the family and I spend one evening pulling salt water taffy, reminds us of the days before all the store bought candies.

We take two cups of sugar, five tablespoons of water a tablespoon of butter, heat it up on the stove till a little dropped from a fork in cold water forms a hard thread, add a tsp. of vanilla and a pinch of cream of tartar then when it cools we sit by the fire and pull and pull until the candy turns white."

Gerald settled himself in a nearby rocking chair, "then" he said, "We wrap the candy in small pieces of wax paper. It was what we had for candies many years ago."

"Course we don't put up the tree until Christmas Eve, reminds me of when we didn't have much more for Christmas than a nicely trimmed tree. We didn't own a vehicle, or a television or a phone."

And, he said, with a twinkle in his fading blue eyes, "We make sure we have a nice sized orange for the toe of the stockings. The orange reminds the missus and me of when we were children; we only had oranges at Christmastime and that orange was always the sweetest juiciest treat of the winter, we sure did savor that orange, making it last all day."

"Are you telling me you try to keep the holidays simple Gerald?"

"Nah, I guess I am just saying for me and the missus the holiday is a time of remembering, we keep things simple during the holidays to help us remember our present day bounty and the blessings over the years."

"Thank You Gerald," I said feeling somewhat lighter, you always have a way of putting things in perspective, Merry Christmas to you.

THE END

THE TRANSFER

By Carolyn Ann Vaughan R.N.

Nightshift 12:01: FRIDAY

: August 23

She plodded to the chart rack, reached for a tissue and wiped at the moisture collecting beneath the collar of her burgundy scrub jacket. Lightly she tapped the button of the ancient desk fan. The tired motor spiked instantly, creating a soft whirring sound.

Every night, shortly after midnight, for the

past two years, before starting her shift, summer or winter, Selma Barclay R.N., turned on the desk fan. The hum of the fan soothed her and shielded her from the blaring, wheezing, sleep noises emanating from the nine elderly, long-term residents of Bentley Psychiatric Ward.

She looked down the darkened hallway and studied the red neon Exit sign. From her place behind the glass of the nursing station she could see the entire length of the ten bed nursing unit.

She hated back shift on the chronic psychiatric ward. She hated the drone of sleeping humanity. She hated the curling bits of yellow paper hanging from the bulletin boards, notices nobody read or removed. But mostly, she hated night shifts.

She'd requested a transfer to day shifts months ago, but her Nursing Supervisor denied her request. She rubbed her hand over tired eyes. For two years now she'd worked the 2300 to 0700 back shift. Sometimes she wondered if she would be able to perform even one more night shift.

Recently she'd begun to fantasize about going into Room 101 and holding a pillow over the face of Alvin MacAroy, a toothless old man who'd been a resident of Bentley Ward for more than fifteen years. In her mind she could see herself, placing the clean white pillow over his face until he ceased his rattling wheezing breath. She wondered if then, the Nursing Supervisor might reconsider a transfer to day shift. Thinking about the pillow brought a smile to her face. Sometimes you just had to think crazy thoughts to get through the night.

<u>04:15</u>

Three hours left in the long and bleary night. Gulping from a red and white thermos standing at her elbow, she felt the hot coffee sting the back of her throat. She'd made her hourly rounds, she'd replenished the Kardex, and checked the drug cupboard, and she'd filed the blood work, and checked to make sure the charts had been signed.

She had caught herself nodding off a time or two, each time jerking upright, startled, disorientated, wondering where or who she was. She wanted to put her head down on the desk and close her eyes, for a minute, just one minute, but she couldn't. She knew she couldn't. She was the only staff member on Bentley ward, the only staff.

The desk fan helped her block out the sleeping sounds, but even the desk fan couldn't block out the wheezing rattle from room 101. For the hundredth time she thanked God for the desk fan. She didn't know what she would do without it.

For the second time Friday night, she wondered what it would be like to go from room to room carrying the pillow, holding the pillow snugly over the face of each piece of sleeping humanity until all the rasping sounds stopped. Dead bodies, quiet dead bodies, soundless people. Maybe then the Nursing Supervisor would take her off night shifts.

She wondered if she was losing it. If maybe she'd been working psych too long. Impatiently she signed her name on each of the charts, Selma Barclay RN, champion of the underdog, defender of the week, always rises to the challenge. They said that once on an evaluation form, but that was years ago. Now she was tired, bone weary tired.

Three more hours tonight and one more night shift tomorrow, then she'd be off for four blessed days. She could do it. She was a nurse. Of course she could do it. Eleven hours total, three tonight eight tomorrow then she would

sleep, really sleep. She could do one more night

shift of course she could.

CHAPTER TWO

(The Transfer)

Evening Shift 21:10 Saturday

Through fogged filled mind, seventeen-year-old runaway, Angel Mason struggled against the bite of hand restraints that dug at her wrists.

"Whoa, child, hold still." The male voice was gentle, soothing.

Angels tongue felt thick. It was an effort to model her words. She wanted to speak to the man, to ask him why her hands were tied to the rail of the bed, but she couldn't get the sounds to form. She thrashed about, pulling from side to side.

"Easy child, there's nothing here to hurt you now."

Angel opened her eyes. The boyish face of a man came into view. He wore a blue linen shirt, a black stethoscope draped about his neck. His nametag identified him as "Beauregard Adams."

Angel fought for memory. She'd been at an all night party out on Long Island beach. She remembered taking a thing called purple microdot. It wasn't the first time she'd tried drugs. But this time the rocks on the beach started to melt and the shadows of the trees along the cliff took on shapes of monsters with horns poised for attack.

"What's happening?" Angel croaked, trying to still a sense of rising panic.

"Must have had a bad acid trip. Don't fight it kid and you'll be back on the streets in less than seventy-two hours."

"Where am I?"

"You're safe." He said. "You're on Bentley Ward, at Island View." And then he added, "the only reason you're on chronic psychiatric is because acute is full." As if it would make any difference to her, which ward she was on.

Angel saw both wrists tied and buckled to silver side rails and the position caused a dull ache between her shoulder blades. "My hands?" she asked, wiggling her fingers.

"It's nothing, just precaution, you were pretty wild when the paramedics brought you in." The mans voice was friendly and warm, but his warmth did nothing to assuage Angel's mounting fear.

"Please," she begged, holding back tears. "Can't you release me?"

"Aw, honey, old Beau here, is just an orderly. But tell you what; if you settle down and get some sleep, I'll leave a note for the night nurse, Selma Barclay. She's a good one she is. Looking mighty tired lately though. Still, I'll tell her you don't cotton to your restraints." He gave Angel's purple spiked hair a fatherly pat and promised to check on her before he went off duty.

"Oh," he added, as an after thought, "don't be alarmed by Betsy over there, she's a little off, harmless though."

Angel could barely see the elderly woman he called Betsy standing very still in the corner of the room holding a raggedy doll. Angel figured Betsy had to be at least eighty, but it was hard to judge. Betsy was the only other patient in the room besides Angel.

For the longest time Betsy stood next to the barred window simply clutching the rag doll to her sagging bosom. "Pretty baby, settle down pretty baby," she crooned to the bit of cloth cradled in her arms.

Faded blue eyes peeked at Angel and the woman seemed to be talking to her, "Get some sleep, it's okay pretty baby." Betsy shuffled towards Angel and flashed a toothless grin. It was then that Angel Mason sought the blessed relief of unconsciousness.

Angel dreamt she was shackled to a tree and a grinning, gaping bear was trying to swallow her whole.

"Angel, Wake up! Wake up! I've brought you some juice." Liza Munroe the evening charge nurse, tried to arouse the new admission.

"No, I, No, I don't want juice." Angel pulled her head away from the plastic straw being pressed against her lips.

"Look miss, it's like this. I have nine old people to attend to and get to bed, most of them senile. You can refuse if you want to, but if I were you, I'd take the juice."

Angel held her ground. "Please, I don't need juice. Just unbuckle me."

"Can't do it honey. I really can't. I don't have a Doctor's order."

Angel focused on the nurse, "but the man, the Doctor was here earlier."

Liza laughed softly. "You must mean Beauregard. He's not a Doctor. What did he tell you?"

Angel kept her tone calm. "He said, if I slept,

the night nurse would take these buckles off my wrists."

"Humph! Selma might remove them when she comes on, but I'm not going to. I told you, I don't have a Doctor's order. And I don't ever, and I mean ever, do anything without a Doctor's order. Now do you want this juice or don't you?"

"No."

"Suit yourself honey. You can refuse."

"I refuse."

"Okey, dokey, but don't go saying I didn't offer you something."

Angel watched as the evening charge nurse wheeled the medication cart over to the old woman who was sitting on the bed still cradling the dirty rag doll.

"Have you been to the toilet, Betsy?"

Angel could see Betsy nod and then as if she were a child and not a wizened old crone she said, "Betsy Flushed, Betsy flushed."

"Good girl! Here then Betsy, here's your sleeping pill and a laxative."

Betsy held out gnarled hands, drank the brown fluid from the little plastic med cup and popped the pill into her gaping slacked jaw. "Sleep pretty baby, sleep."

"Yes dear. You sleep, but first let me fix your panties."

Angel watched as the nurse adjusted the

plastic underwear, pulling it snug over brown wrinkled skin. "You don't want to have a messy bum, now do you, that will just make work for Selma."

Betsy pulled back. "Selma bad mommy! Selma bad mommy!"

"Tut, now Betsy, you know you can't say that."

The charge nurse shot Angel an apologetic look. "I don't know what's gotten into her, for the last few months or so Betsy has been calling Selma a bad mommy."

The nurse looked at Angel and made a circling sign with her finger to her head, and whispered, "cuckoo you know."

For the first time since she'd been admitted to this bizarre world, Angel Mason laughed. Not because the nurse was making cuckoo signs. But because she could see the old woman mimicking the gesture while the nurses back was turned.

Angel decided if she was going to spend the night tied to her bed in a mental ward she'd better find out who Betsy was. She felt kind of sorry for the old lady, having to wear a diaper and all. Angel had learned enough living on the streets the past few years to know it made more sense to make friends than to look for enemies.

"That's a pretty doll Betsy. Can you bring it closer so I can see it?"

The old woman shuffled forward until she

stood a few paces from Angel's bed. Tentatively the old women reach out and gingerly poked the top of Angel's spiked purple hair. "Oh, pretty baby," she said. Patting first Angel's hair and then what was left of the yellow wool of the rag doll.

Betsy's eyes grew wide as she saw Angel's wrists restrained by the buckle straps. Her wizened old face began to crumple and Angel thought Betsy was about to cry. "Oh poor baby, poor baby," Betsy said, running dry warm fingers over Angels wrists.

Angel held her breath, barely daring to make a motion. "Betsy," she whispered. "Do you think you could undo my hand?"

CHAPTER THREE

(The Transfer)

At first, Angel thought Betsy hadn't heard, because the old woman continued to croon, "poor baby, poor baby." But gently Betsy placed the rag doll on the sheets of Angel's bed and began to work bony fingers beneath the buckle of the wrist restraint.

Angel dared not move for fear the old woman

would lose concentration. Angel saw the little flap holding the buckle begin to loosen, a fraction at first, but slowly, painstakingly, Betsy worked at it until there was a loop about an inch high.

"Betsy, You get away from there!" Betsy jumped and Angel felt her own hot blinding tears of frustration gather beneath her eyelids.

Beauregard swooped into the room grasped Betsy by the shoulders, plucked the rag doll from Angels bed and guided Betsy back to her side of the room. Betsy began to whimper, a soft mewing sound.

"Oh, come on Sweets, Daddy's not mad. Now come on Betsy, get into bed." Betsy began to croon to her dolly, "poor baby, poor baby."

Beauregard turned towards Angel, his dark face a mask of controlled anger. "You had no right to encourage her like that. The poor old soul doesn't like restraints. God knows she's had more than enough of them in her day."

"Well I..."

"I know you just wanted to be rid of em. But like I told you already, Selma will probably remove them when she comes on duty. She's been known to bend a rule a little." He reached behind Angels head and handed her a cord with a button at the end of it, then he placed it in the palm of her hand so that even with the wrist restrains in place she would be able to signal the nursing station.

"Now you do as I say, and you'll make this

whole experience a little easier on your self. It's almost change of shift. You wait for a half hour or so, give Selma a chance to listen to report and read her notes and then give her a buzz, if you talk real nice to her, I suspect she might just take off your hand restraints. Especially if you promise her you won't make a peep the rest of the night. Liza and I are going off duty now, so you wait a bit and then call her. Understood?"

Angel nodded her head. This was one helluva place she'd landed herself in and it seemed to have rules she didn't understand. "Thanks mister, I'll do as you say."

"Smart girl," he said, as he winked and left the room.

Angel decided she'd wait at least an hour before she buzzed the night nurse, no point in getting her pissed.

CHAPTER FOUR

(The Transfer)

<u>Night Shift 24:00: Saturday,</u>

Selma Barclay slipped the taped report into the machine and listened while Liza Munroe's voice droned on about the events of the evening "Liza Munroe, recording for evenings."

Who else would be recording, Selma wondered, Santa Claus?

"Ward census nine plus one."

Now that was something different, plus one, an admission to chronic?

"Jake Reardon was incontinent twice."

As if Selma cared how many times the old guy wet himself.

"Betsy Turner was given a laxative."

When wasn't Betsy given a laxative? Selma leafed through the notes left by the orderly.

Beau had written in heavy bold script, that the new admit wanted her wrist restraints removed, beside it he wrote in bold letters, NO ORDER.

Selma pulled the new patient's chart. Sure enough, there were no doctors' orders to remove restraints. She scanned through the data. The poor kid, she was just a runaway getting herself into trouble, been seen in Emerg by the admitting Doctor, guy probably wrote hand restraints to keep the emergency room nurses happy. Then the kid had been shipped off to chronic psych. The ER Doc probably expected the kid to end up on the short stay psych unit; too bad short term was full.

Selma searched the chart, she saw that the ward psychiatrist Dr. Blaine had telephoned in verbal admission orders, said he'd see the patient in the morning at his regular rounds, his verbal orders were mostly routine stuff, blood work, diet. Hadn't said a word about wrist restraints.

The old coot probably didn't know the kid

was still wearing wrist restraints. Selma wouldn't go down the hall to remove them, just yet, she still had her paper work to do, but if the kid was awake when she made her first round, what the hell she'd take them off. You had to do something now and then on night shifts to let administration know you were alive, otherwise they forgot all about you.

CHAPTER FIVE

(The Transfer)

Selma snapped the off button of the tape recorder. There was no point in listening to the rest of the drivel. Nothing ever changed on chronic.

She was tired, so very tired, and the snoring sounds from Room 101 seemed louder than she could ever remember. She placed her hands over ears trying to block out the constant whining wheeze.

Suddenly without warning the desk fan above her head stopped and when it stopped Selma felt roar emanating from Room 101. It was as though a drone of helicopters had entered the ward.

Quietly and deliberately Selma closed the orderlies notebook. Without the fan, Alvin's snore clawed at Selma's soul like razors along the soft underbelly of a robin.

Soundlessly, Selma walked, as only a night nurse can, into the darkened room just off the nurses station. She paused for a moment. She noticed the hearing aid and the false teeth sitting on the bedside table. Beau should have put those teeth in a denture cup. She thought.

The room smelled faintly of a dirty urinal. Her foot caught on the over bed table. She steadied herself. The pillow was in the Geri chair by Alvin's bed, just as for months she'd imagined it would be. Consciously, deliberately, she picked up the pillow with both hands.

Alvin MacAvoy lay flat on his back, his skinny chest heaving rhythmically. A string of spittle curled down over his lip and bubbled with each screech of his breath. She advanced slowly towards him until the sound of his wheezy, shrieking sleep noises thundered in her ears like the roar of a thousand fire trucks.

As her eyes adjusted to the darkened room, she saw three silver nose hairs protruding from his right nostril. Beau should have trimmed those. She held the pillow to her body like a shield against the clatter of Alvin's sleeps noises while she moved in closer. When the pillow was within inches of his wrinkled brown cheeks, she placed it firmly over his face.

Alvin struggled once, Selma exerted more pressure. Alvin tried to get bony fingers beneath the pillow. Selma held on. Alvin MacAvoy jerked his scrawny legs making a feeble scissor cut. Finally, the wheezy, shrieking sleep noises ceased and Selma found peace. Selma counted slowly to sixty. One little rabbit, two little rabbits...

Selma replaced the pillowcase with a fresh one and gently returned the pillow to the Geri chair. Alvin would need his pillow when the day shift came in to take him for a walk. Alvin's backside always got sore if he didn't have his pillow to sit on.

She straightened Alvin's top sheet so it lay neatly just below his jaw and wiped a bloody string of spittle from his chin. She kissed the small St. Christopher medal hanging about her neck. She was glad Alvin's wheeze was better tonight. Come to think of it she couldn't remember a night shift when Alvin's piercing wheeze hadn't grated on her nerves.

Selma left the room and quietly closed the door. She smoothed her hands down over her uniform and plucked at imaginary pieces of lint. Something didn't seem right to her, but she didn't quite know what it was. She had to get off nights. She just had to.

She turned towards the nursing station when she caught the blink of the call light at the end of the corridor. Why did she have this uneasy feeling in the pit of her stomach?

Selma opened the room occupied by Betsy and the new Admission.

CHAPTER SIX

(The Transfer)

Shortly after Beau left her alone with Betsy, Angel had dozed. She was awakened by the distant sounds of a shrill wheezing sound, but a few moments later the sound stopped. It was dark out yet the glow from the outside parking lot lit up the shadows on the far wall. Betsy had fallen asleep and Angel found the wrists restraints becoming more and more uncomfortable.

Tentatively she pressed the buzzer Beau had given her. She had rehearsed what she would say when the night nurse came in. It wasn't as if she were actually a psychiatric patient. She had simply taken some bad drugs. Not too smart maybe and even illegal but not crazy.

Angel felt the door to her room opening and a woman with short-cropped brown hair turned on the overhead light. If Angel could have leapt from the bed and hid in the closet she would have done so. Never in her life had she ever been so utterly petrified.

The nurse wore a nametag, the same kind Beau had worn. But, it was the woman's eyes that terrified Angel. The eyes were dark and hooded with a glassy look. There were smoldering dark circles under the eyes and Angel was certain the woman didn't know where she was. Angel had seen that vacant look many times on the streets. Always she avoided people with eyes like that. Angel was beyond sorry she had rung her buzzer.

Angel heard Betsy whimper. The nurse, with the killer look in her eyes, whipped her head around toward the sound and sniffed at the air. Angel could smell the distinct odour of feces. Betsy must have dirtied her diaper. The nurse moved swiftly, pulled a pillow from beneath the old woman's head and with cool and deliberate action she placed the pillow over Betsy's face and continued to hold.

CHAPTER SEVEN

(The Transfer)

<u>TWO WEEKS LATER:</u>

It's been two weeks since Betsy's death. Angel no longer wears wrist restraints but she doesn't' say much anymore, just "sleep pretty baby, sleep" and sometimes Angel mutters, "bad mommy, bad mommy."

Beauregard and the evening Charge Nurse,

Liza Munroe, occasionally discuss what a shame it was Betsy's death happened the same night Angel Mason was admitted.

"Imagine the poor kid coming up with a story about Selma smothering poor old Betsy."

It was Beau that said, "guess two deaths in one night, the restraints and bad street drugs must have completely unhinged the poor kid. Too bad, I surely do hope she eventually recovers. She was a nice kid."

Selma Barclay RN doesn't work night shifts at Island Pacific psychiatric anymore. Her request for a temporary transfer to day shift finally came through. She stayed another week but then she received an opportunity to work on the children's unit at Mercy Hospital on the lower East side.

Selma bumped into Beau one evening at the movie theatre. When he asked her how she liked her new job she told him she'd really enjoyed it at first, but lately she had to put in for another transfer, she said they had shifted her to night work again. She said she just hated to hear the poor little children crying all night long. Said it just about drove her to distraction.

THE END

CRYING IN

CHURCH

By Carolyn Ann Vaughan RN

(Nurses Diary page summer 2015)

Last Sunday, while sitting in church, I encountered the most mysterious and confusing of experiences. As the small congregation began to sing an old hymn, one

I've heard many times before, "Just as I am, without one plea" my eyes filled with tears until I could barely read the hymnbook. My tears came unannounced, unbidden, and mysteriously, but mostly my tears embarrassed me.

Why was I crying? It was only a song. I was not in any form of crisis. My world was safe, yet I wept, and the weeping confused me. Fortunately, I found a tissue in my handbag and inconspicuously wiped the tears from my face.

After a time, I gained control and the service came to an end. As I left the pew, I spoke briefly to a stranger, and the stranger asked me to write the words of another short tune customarily sung at the beginning of the service. The tune begins with "Lord listen to your children praying"

The stranger said the words had moved her, and would I write them for her. She explained she had difficulty holding a pen. I of course wrote out the few lines because she asked for my help.

For the rest of the day, my mind drifted back to my tears in the church. And as I pondered, I recalled times in my life when I've worn a brave face though feeling emotionally bruised. I remembered times when I've struggled to rise above perceived hurts or been overwhelmed with my workload, and felt my angers, fearful of admitting, "I hurt, please help me."

Somewhere in late afternoon, I concluded, like it or not, (and frankly I didn't) that I have at times been emotionally needy. A person who has yearned for the acceptance of others, even worked hard to gain acceptance. But I had to face the truth. I have seldom simply asked for acceptance, but instead have struggled to attain it. Always be the strong Nurse, in control able and capable. I finally decided one of the reason for my tears was that the song spoke of acceptance, "just as I am", not perfect, maybe even conflicted and confused, but still valued.

I considered this new found knowledge and wondered about the truth of it. Was I valuable, not because I'd worked to gain approval, but simply because I was.

Then at the end of my day as I sat down to write this diary page, I remembered the stranger who requested my help. I began to wonder if perhaps, along with my tears, she too was teaching me something. Was it possible that acceptance, approval, and even help were available simply by asking? I felt as though I were on the doorstep of a lesson in personal insight.

Someone once said all life is a mystery. I'm not sure about life, but I know trying to understand self is a challenge. I've not yet come to a complete understanding of the why, of my tears in the church service, but I believe I can agree with Miss Charlotte Elliott who penned the words to the hymn, "Just as I am, Without One Plea" there is tremendous comfort in believing I am valued not because I've gained perfection, or even because I've worked hard to earn acceptance, but because I'm willing to believe I am treasured and that help is available, simply for the asking.

THE END

LYDIA'S FOLLY

Preamble:

Lydia Silver is a top-notch nurse but her personal life is in shambles. She believed her dream of having a child died the night her paramedic fiancé Jake Boutlier flipped his ambulance on the twisting Coastal highway. She believed this, until the last night of the health convention in Toronto when in a moment of desperation she made the decision that would change her life forever.

LYDIA'S FOLLY

By Carolyn Ann Vaughan R.N.

"Are you crazy? Are you completely insane?"

"Well I..."

"Oh for heavens sakes Lydia, nobody sleeps with a stranger, just to have a baby."

Shelly McKenzie stirred vigorously at the fish chowder she was preparing for the church supper. "Do you even know his name?"

"Well, of course I know his name," said her sister Lydia, "its Duncan Mark Fanshawe, M. D."

Lydia repeated the name, "Duncan Mark

Fanshawe, M.D." as if knowing the strangers name might somehow make her actions more acceptable.

Lydia riffled trembling fingers through dark curly hair, "Shelly it didn't mean anything. A one night stand at the health convention in Toronto last weekend. You know there's never been anyone for me but Jake."

Shelly McKenzie closed her eyes and drew a deep breath. "Jake is dead Lydia! Nothing, not even a stranger's baby, can bring him back."

Lydia's eyes filled with tears. "I know he's dead Shelly I've known it everyday for the past six months." Lydia swallowed a mouthful of cold coffee. "But, I have to go on living and I honestly don't know how I can do that."

Lydia swiped a renegade tear threatening to slide down her cheek. "There's never been any man in my life but Jake. Now there never will be." Lydia's voice sounded younger than her thirty-two years. "No one was hurt Shelly. No one! It's not like I'll ever see Duncan Fanshawe again."

Lydia loved her older sister. She was the only family she had left. And she didn't want to argue with her. "Besides," she said, "who knows, maybe I'm not even pregnant."

Shelly's face brightened. "Saints preserve us. I honestly hope your not. It was a crazy idea Lydia. I've never known you to act so rashly."

Lydia finished helping her sister bottle up the chowder. Perhaps she shouldn't have confided in her sister until she knew for sure. But she had to tell someone or bust. And Shelly was more than her sister. Shelly was her best friend.

"Do you think I've made enough?" Shelly asked, ladling the last of the chowder into two five-gallon jars.

Lydia smiled to herself. Shelly always worried about taking enough food to church suppers. "Oh, Shelly not even your crew can finish up all this chowder."

Lydia's sister pushed a wisp of blond hair from her face" You know how Andrew, Luke and Josh pack away the grub, I just like to be sure."

"I'm sure Shelly there's enough chowder here

to feed all of Sheet Harbour."

Lydia laughed. "Not that Sheet Harbour has a <u>lot</u> of folks to worry about feeding. You can put the whole population of the town in a medium sized city block."

Shelly wiped the lids of the jars with a clean towel before applying a seal and looked quizzically at her sister. "You know Lydia I've often wondered why you came back. It isn't as if you couldn't make a life for yourself in Halifax, or Toronto or Montreal even. All the big city hospitals are crying for nurses, with your experience they'd snap you up in a minute."

Lydia placed the jars in a carton and added the rolls her sister had baked the day before. "I love this place Shelly. It's my home. And the cottage on the ocean Dad left me is absolutely perfect. "Besides," she added teasingly, "the cottage is a good place to raise a child or two."

Her sister gave her a quick tap with the dishtowel. "Honest to God Lydia your determined spirit is going to get you in over your head one of these days. I just feel it. You know what gram always said. 'Roosters always come home to roost' not that I ever really understood what she meant by that. By the way, are you coming to the church supper tonight?"

"No, I have night shift at the hospital."

"Yuk, how many night shifts do you have this time?"

Lydia wiped her hands on the tea towel "Two weeks worth. It was the trade off for going to the medical convention in Toronto. You know the convention where maybe I did and maybe I didn't manage to become pregnant." She said because she couldn't really help teasing her sister.

******

At ten minutes to eight Lydia rushed through the automatic doors of Melway Hospital just as Mary Delmonte and Rena Ogilvie, two of the Day shift nurses were stepping off the elevator. "Heh Mary' how is it?" Lydia asked.

Mary Delmonte rolled her eyes and gave

a wave. "It's been the Q word."

Lydia smiled to herself. Nobody on hospital staff ever said the ward was quiet. It was an unwritten hospital rule. To actually say the <u>quiet</u> word was to open the floodgates to the outpatients department. Then you'd be swamped until midnight. Lydia breathed a sigh of relief. "Great," she responded, "just what I need, a few easy shifts."

Mary called out to her. "Sharon's already waiting in the report room for you and I think Dr. Henry Wallows is on call."

Lydia groaned as she opened the door to the report room. Doc Wallows was the on call physician. He is one of the older Doctors and hated to be disturbed after midnight. Not that

Lydia could really blame Henry Wallows for not wanting to take call. Heaven knows with all the hours the two town physicians put in, it was amazing they hadn't left years ago. But Sheet Harbour had a way of growing on a person.

Lydia stepped into the report room and hung her navy fleece jacket on the hook. Sharon Andrews was seated at the table. The tape recorder, the patient Kardex and a paper and pencil lay on the table in front of her.

"Say how was your convention? You did go to the health care seminar in Toronto last week didn't you?"

Lydia felt the heat rising in her cheeks. "It was good," she mumbled, avoiding eye contact, and I hope productive she thought remembering her last night at the conference. Lydia wasn't the sort to go for a one-night stand but she missed her fiancé terribly and she desperately wanted a child She highly doubted she would ever find another love, but she knew she could love a child.

Melway Hospital is small, only twenty active nursing beds. When Lydia first came to Melway, she'd been sure it would be a laid back nursing job. But the rural setting was more challenging than she had expected.

It was not just the in-patients she and Sharon would have to be concerned about. It was also the outpatient dept. On a good night, she and her co-worker would go through the night routine dealing with only the problems of the ward. On a difficult night, they would have to contend with one, two, or maybe even five outpatients. That was the problem with outpatients it was unpredictable.

"Do you want to do inpatient or out?" Sharon asked, holding the keys to the inpatient medication cupboard in her hands.

Lydia shrugged, "I think I'll take outpatients, I've been off for two weeks"

Sharon pocketed the keys and tapped the play button on the tape recorder. The two nurses concentrated on the taped report given by Mary Delmonte. Mary's voice was crisp, clear, matter of fact.

"Current census fourteen, room three, Alvin Mason, 72-year-old patient of Dr. Wallows, admitted Nov. fifth with diagnosis of post-op repair of left hip fracture."

Lydia looked up from her notepaper. "When did he break his hip?" she asked.

Sharon pressed the pause button on the tape recorder and flipped through the Kardex until she found Room three, "says he fell off his porch step on Oct 31. They repaired it that night at the Queen Elizabeth Hospital in Halifax and then kept him for five days."

Lydia placed a tiny check mark beside Alvin's name. She would have to make sure he had pillows between his legs so as not to compromise the repair work. "Has he been ambulating?"

Sharon nodded. "No, he doesn't like getting

out of bed, but we really should try to get him moving"

Sharon resumed the taped message. Mary's voice continued. "Please ambulate with assistance times two, non insulin dependent diabetic, medicated with Tylenol # 3, times two, oh I almost forgot, he's requesting a laxative. Not sure what he uses at home you'll have to ask." Lydia wrote lax beside Alvin's name although it wouldn't be her job to give him any laxatives. Sharon was medication nurse for the ward, but with only two nurses on the floor, Lydia and Sharon were required to act as a team.

Mary's voice continued, "Room four, vacant. Room five Bessie Johnson, 93, patient of Dr.

Wallows, awaiting nursing home placement, no change." Lydia wrote Bessie's name on her slip of paper but wrote nothing beside it. Bessie had been in hospital for over two months there really was nothing new to say about her. All the staff was familiar with Bessie and the care she required.

"Room six vacant. Room seven new admission, Tiffany Benson, 7, patient of Dr. Caruthers, admitted today, gastroenteritis, NPO" Lydia scribbled nothing to eat beside Tiffany's name. "Vomiting times two, diarrhea times one. IV Ringers Lactate on the pump at 100 cc an hour, 300 cc TBA" Lydia made a note to check Tiffany's IV before three hours were up. "IV Gravol at 1600 hours, no further vomiting since that time."

Lydia glanced up from her paper. "Is Tiffany Benson, Gail's daughter?" Gail Benson was one of the Registered Nurses who did relief work, usually on weekends.

"Yes."

"Is Gail planning on spending the night?"

"No, she has two little ones at home."

Lydia put a star beside Tiffany's name, knowing she was Gail's daughter might be helpful in drawing the child out."

Mary's crisp clear voice continued giving details regarding the other five inpatients. Both Sharon and Lydia scribbled brief notes about the patients on their pieces of paper, then folded the paper lengthwise, and slipped their papers into the pocket of their scrub uniforms. Both nurses would consult the paper more than once during their twelve-hour shift, sometimes to find a piece of data, sometimes to scribble pertinent information to be passed on in the morning to day shift.

"You want to pass night lunches while I pour my bedtime medications?" Sharon asked.

"Sure, it'll give me a chance to see some of the new faces I don't know yet. I'll check the Doctors orders for you too if you want." Both nurses understood passing night lunch and checking Doctors orders was the inpatient nurses job, but they always worked as a team.

They really could use an extra pair of hands on nights, but with the geographical location of

Melway Hospital, it was unlikely they would ever have extra staff. The closest hospital in their district was a two-hour drive along the twisting, winding coastal road. Two hours in summer, in winter, it could easily be three and attracting nurses to the rural hospital was always a challenge.

Lydia grabbed the tray of night lunches from the fridge, she checked to make sure there was at least one diabetic snack for Alvin.

She could hear the clink of the mop as the night maintenance man mopped up the seating area surrounding the outpatient waiting room. "Heh Joe," she asked, "get your deer yet?"

Joe was getting close to retirement. He was great with all the nursing staff. Treated them like his daughters. His one passion other than the hospital was hunting.

"Nah, Lydia, but I seed the tracks, big buck, real big buck, all I guts to do is catch it. How'd the big city treat ya?"

"Great Joe! Great!" Lydia could feel herself blushing, if only he knew.

"Guess I'd better pass night lunches."

"You's two want coffee later?" Joe would bring them a strong pot of coffee and even a snack or two from the cafeteria sometime after midnight just before he finished his work and locked the hospital up tight for the night.

"Sure Joe, coffee would be great, and maybe a piece of lemon pie if there's any left over."

Lydia asked hopefully.

Melway used to be a bigger hospital with room for forty-five in-patients. Medical staff once performed surgical procedures, delivered babies, but with the closing of the fisheries and the retirement of Melway's only surgeon, the Provincial Health board downsized Melway to ten active inpatient beds, upped the day clinic practice and used the extra room in the hospital to give the two remaining doctors office space. Serious cases where stabilized at Melway and then sent via helicopter to Halifax. Less serious cases went in by ambulance.

Lydia checked her tray and selected the diabetic snack the kitchen had sent up for Alvin and entered his room. The one positive about the downsizing of the hospital was that most rooms were now privates. It was rare when a patient had to share a room with a fellow patient. The man that lay on the bed in front of her had a shock of white hair and bearded stubble. "Say you old codger how did you ever break your hip?" She asked.

Alvin's watery blue eyes twinkled, "Well, me and the missus, was handing out treats to the ghosts and goblins," he rubbed his hand across his grizzled face, "next thing you knows I was sitting on me butt. Hurt like the dickens it did."

Lydia passed him his nighttime snack. "I'll bet it did. You go in by ambulance or by chopper?"

"Doc Wallows sent me in by road, darn worse

ride I's ever had, almost broke me other hip."

Lydia chuckled, "I've heard it's a rough old road in the back of an ambulance, Jake always said," Lydia felt the catch in her breath and a misty film of water gathering beneath her lashes, it seemed like every time she turned around she was recalling something Jake always said. Would she ever be able to put his death behind her?

Alvin activated the control on his bed so he was sitting almost upright. "You miss that lad don't ya Lydia? He was a good lad was Jake. Durn shame when he and Johnny flipped their ambulance, but that's a bad curve there at Ship Harbour, real bad curve."

Lydia walked over to the bed and activated

the controls so that Alvin was sitting no more than 45 degrees upright. "You know you shouldn't have your bed up so high Alvin, at least not until your hip heals."

Her words were blunt, harsher than she intended. What was the matter with her anyway? Jake was gone. Gone. Oh, why hadn't they gotten married? Why hadn't they started a family? She loved her job, she loved her town, but she was lonely, achingly lonely. Her sister was right. She must be insane. Having sex with a stranger.

Duncan Mark Fanshawe MD he wasn't a stranger he was Duncan Mark Fanshawe. Oh Lydia don't kid yourself, you hardly knew him. A stranger, a face even now, she couldn't recall.

When she'd gone with him to his room the last night of the conference, it was Jakes voice she heard. It was Jake's caress she felt.

Lydia finished passing out the night lunches to the rest of the in-patients and then checked the on call registry for the weekend. It was at that point that she thought her heart might stop beating. "D.M. Fanshawe MD." She could barely catch her breath. This couldn't be happening. It was impossible. Her voice trembled as she held the shaking paper out to Sharon. "What do you know about this she crowed? Stabbing the paper under Sharon's nose. Who is D.M. Fanshawe MD?"

Sharon continued to drop pills into plastic medicine cups. "Just what it says I guess. D.M.

Fanshawe MD. He's the new locum coming to cover for Henry Wallows.

Lydia stilled her racing heart. There had to be a million D. M. Fanshaws well maybe not a million but at least a few across the country. It was a hoax, a cruel joke. Lydia could barely speak through dusty lips. "Do you know where he's from?" She asked, trying to quell the panic arising in her voice.

"Lydia for goodness sakes, you look as if you've seen a ghost, he's just a locum we've had a number of them over the years. Toronto I think? Why? Do you know him?"

Lydia could feel the floor swaying beneath her. "No, I, uh, I..."

"Oh well, you'll have a chance to meet him

tomorrow night. He's working the weekend." Sharon finished putting the pills in separate cubicles. "I guess Henry's going to take the opportunity to visit his grandchildren. Heard the new guys quite a hunk though."

Lydia shuffled the papers around. What kind of mess had she gotten herself into? She'd purposely chosen a stranger so she'd have no entanglements. She didn't believe in fate. She believed people chose their own futures.

Truth is, she didn't believe she'd ever run across him again, she had just been so achingly lonely.

She managed to finish the rest of the night shift concentrating solely on the duties of the ward. Fortunately the night shift ended routinely.

*****

She slept fitfully during the day, waking and dozing, waking and dozing by the time her alarm went off she thought she'd gone ten rounds with a heavy weight boxer.

If she hadn't just come back off vacation she might have called in sick, she certainly felt queasy enough. She did not want to meet the new locum, DM Fanshaw MD, she most certainly did not.

THE END

TO BE CONTINUED......

EUTHANASIA

HOW SHALL YOU DIE?

By Carolyn Ann Vaughan RN

For years I have struggled with euthanasia. Euthanasia is a word taken from the Greek language meaning "good death" in today's world, euthanasia has come to mean, "action taken" to achieve a good death, some might call this assisted suicide, or physician assisted suicide, others like Derek Humphrey, a journalist and author of the book "Final Exit" would call it "self deliverance."

My concern is deeply personal. I hold conflicting feelings about death. I don't believe in the death penalty. I was twelve years old when the last two men were hanged in Canada. The year was 1962. Fourteen years later in 1976 Canada abolished the death penalty. I believe this was a step of compassion directed towards one group of peoples. I believe a number of persons who would have been hanged had we still practiced the art of Government hanging who have since been exonerated by DNA testing, must also be grateful for collective compassion. So while I do not believe in the death penalty, I do believe people have the right to active euthanasia.

In 1984, I was a nurse of one year when the government finally permitted a "Do Not Resuscitate" order to be placed on a medical chart. Prior to this time, I was advised by my Catholic Head Nurse and the Catholic Institution which employed me, to "walk slowly nurse, walk slowly" when confronted with applying heroic measures for individuals who stood at deaths door and living held no hope of quality of life, in other words do as little as you possible could to intervene with the dying process. I recall a study saying nurses avoided the rooms of the dying, I suspect they were following the "walk slowly nurse, walk slowly."

While our Country abolished death by hanging in 1976, almost forty years later it has yet to address the issues of compassion for those facing the final journey or being tortuously afflicted in times of illness or disease.

Why is this? Is it because we are cowardly? Is it because we are willing to allow the medical profession to ease death "wink, wink" by massive doses of narcotics, yet we handcuff, chastise and threaten to imprison a doctor who chooses to administer heart stopping nitroglycerine and sodium chloride when the "wink, wink" method goes horribly awry.

Do we fail to address the issue of "self

deliverance" because someone, somewhere, gleans a profit should we linger in our dying? Is it because we do not personally face life and death issues on a daily basis? Is it because the "dying hard people" pass on without voice so we can avoid addressing the issues as long as humanly possible.

Is it because we are afraid to face our own personal death, therefore we have delayed compassion? I do not know the answers to these questions.

Did we sanctioned abortion and the abolition of the Canadian death penalty because we could sooth our collective conscience. Say, "abortion doesn't really affect me, and those sentenced to die for a crime don't really affect me" so reluctantly we made laws about these issues, but death due to illness and disease, yes that could affect me, therefore we choose to delay an answer.

We have chosen to uphold the abolition of the death penalty. We have chosen to permit abortion. We have even prided ourselves as a nation slow to war, yet we come so leisurely to a resolution regarding how to deal with death from illness, disease and tortuous living.

Instead, we laid this enormous burden upon the modern health care profession, and abandoned to the luck or non-luck of the dying individual for a good death.

Our grandparents did not have this issue, they did not have the technology to keep the dying alive beyond the point, nor did they possess any procedures needed to keep the "barely alive" heart beating.

To compound our action of failing to make a collective decision we abandoned, to a ten-year prison term, Robert Latimer the father who could not bear to see his daughter suffer one more medical procedure. I believe our collective cowardice has refused to remember that death is the final resting place of each of us. Death is.

I believe Dr. Henry Morgentaler was a courageous man, steadfast in his resolve to provide women with choice. I don't believe in unwanted neglected and abused infants nor traumatized women being forced to deliver.

Before the right to safe Physician assisted abortions, society sued, jailed and fire bombed his clinics. Still he persevered; he was a compassionate man who believed in a woman's choice.

I don't believe in War. I believe it is an intrinsically flawed method of conflict resolution. I don't believe in death inflicted for the sake of war. But I do believe in choice.

So, what can I say about active euthanasia, and why do I say it? I say, I agree with the people of the state of Oregon, who in 1997 passed a law called "Death with Dignity Act." Under this act, an adult suffering from a terminal illness was allowed by law to receive a prescription from his physician in consultation with a secondary physician, and allowed to take oral medications leading to their own death.

A physician or health care practitioner was not allowed to administer the medication, only the patient themselves could self-administer. I do not think this law addressed all the issues needed for compassion when it comes to the dying process, or a good death.

Some stats from the beginning of the Oregon law:

1997 at that time 10 persons received a prescription 8 persons used it.

1998 (first full year) 23 persons received a prescription 15 used it.

1999 -33 persons received a prescription and

27 used it.

2000 -39 persons received a prescription 27 used it.

2001 -44 persons received a prescription and 21 persons used it.

2002 −58 persons received a prescription 38 used it.

2003 −67 persons 42 used it. (Oregon State Cancer Act)

Dr. Kevorkian, who also did not believe the law went far enough served eight years in prison for assisting others to die" he said "Death is not a Crime"

Oregon didn't get it right will Canada? I believe Canada is on the path towards physician-assisted suicide (euthanasia) , and I say it is about time.

What do the Oregon State Figures say to me? They say although some requested the oral prescription not all chose to use it. I suspect some felt they wanted to live their life until the end. I suspect they wanted the assurance that if the end became too hard they could opt out. I know I would want that choice for myself.

Would I want to take my own life? Of course not. Would I choose to die by my own hand, if I were unable to emotionally, and physically continue – absolutely! One of the most horrendous issues concerning my own brush with cancer in 1994 was the feeling of complete lack of personal control. And if I, a nurse, able to voice my needs to colleagues, with a supportive and loving family, could feel this devastating loss of control, how much more so must the person confronted by the medical system at their time of dying, feel this total loss of control. How much more helpless must a father feel in the face of excruciating suffering of his child?

The Oregon State "Death with Dignity Act" did not address all the issues surrounding dying, but it did provide a measure of personal control to those in Oregon. However it did not benefit those in other states. How cruel is this? I once nursed a patient who did not live in Oregon and who decided to use methods described in the death book "Final Exit" I believe these were similar methods used by

Robert Latimer when his young daughter Tracey's life became unbearable.

Just recently, the province of Quebec has permitted a hospice to move towards physician-assisted euthanasia as part of end of life health care. Canada is in the process of accepting physician-assisted euthanasia as a part of health care. I say it is about time. I also ask if Canada will be courageous enough to come to the aid of others in need of a compassionate and caring death. I sincerely hope so.

Whether we like it or not, each of us, (and yes, that includes you) at one time or another, will be called upon to face our own death or the death of a loved one, therefore we all, everyone of us, has a stake in this issue.

Will Canada's new law be a benefit to the Latimer family, where the Saskatchewan, father of four, chose to end the tortuous life of his daughter Tracey? I sincerely hope so it is the humane thing to do, instead, Robert Latimer served a prison term from 1993 until full day parole in 2010, for being unable to subject his child to one more tortuous medical intervention. Will the act of Euthanasia be available to children like Tracey?

Will Canada's new law be of benefit to people such as the American girl, Karen Ann Quinlan, who following an ingestion of tranquilizers and alcohol in 1975, lived ten years, in coma, on tube feedings, in a nursing home, after the removal of a mechanical ventilator. The tragedy of the Quinlan family led to what is now called a living will or advanced directives. Karen died one year after Canada finally allowed the Do Not Resuscitate order to be placed on medical charts.

And what about the agonizing dying hours of a Halifax patient and the months of trauma sustained by his female physician, Dr. Nancy Morrison, initially charged with his murder because she chose to administer a potentially lethal injection of nitroglycerin and potassium chloride when narcotics and any other comfort measures failed to relieve his horrors. (Dr. Morrison was found not guilty of murder and charges were dropped.)

Will the new Canadian law be of assistance to people like Sue Rodriguez, a forty–two year old mother who while dying of Lou Gehrig's disease petitioned the supreme court of Canada, under Charter rights for assisted suicide. Sue's petition was denied by a vote of five to four. She died in 1994 and although we are creeping towards addressing the issue we have not yet done so.

We have not yet fully addressed the right to a physician-assisted death. I hope moving forward Canada will be brave enough to act on death with dignity, and make such a process available to those who choose this and to those who need and deserve this. Death is not the enemy, nor an unnatural process. Death is the final journey for each and every single one of us.

Not all death is painful and contorted; many times death is peaceful and quiet, and I thank God for this, but one thing is an absolute positive. Death is.

The problem of course is not that death is, the problem is that medical science, can now seriously impair the natural death process. Either through surgeries (that sometimes go awry) or through machines, tubes and feeding methods that keep a body alive while the mind and spirit become trapped in a vacuum and the body is left to slowly work its way towards a fetal position and in some cases such as Tracey Latimer's suffer agonizing unrelieved torture just by living.

Terry Shiavo, a Florida woman, was denied the natural death that would accompany her condition from 1990 until 2005. For fifteen years, a court and legal battle raged between her husband who sought removal of a feeding apparatus and her parents, who hoping for an eventual miracle fought for keeping the feeding apparatus. My heart ached for them all. Such is medical science, but is a prolonged death of fifteen years ethical, or is it instead the cruelty of medical science.

What do I want for me? For this is the only way I can truly relate to this issue. I want to die with peace and dignity. Free of pain, BUT if this is not possible, I want to know I can take charge of my death as I see fit. In addition, if I want this for myself, how can I in good conscience not want this for another soul who may be unlucky enough to die horrendously, or be trapped in a dying process taking fifteen years.

What about you, how shall you die? In Canada, the question is still unresolved. On February 6, 2015, the Supreme Court of Canada ruled unanimously that the law banning assisted suicide was unconstitutional. Canada remains in limbo. We can still be more humane to our pets than we can to our population. Where is justice, where is compassion?

THE END

THE JAGGED

EDGE

By Carolyn Ann Vaughan RN

There was no reason to believe terror trampled in the park. It was a wondrous fall day, maple trees had taken on an orange glow, the scent of the air held a hint of fall and afternoon sun still shone with a gentle warmth picking out golden highlights in the swinging pony tail of the young woman running. It was the highlights in her long blond tresses that attracted his attention.

Alana had just started a new job as Director of the Children's Aquatic Centre teaching swimming lessons to special needs kids. She hoped by taking the job for a few years she'd be able to save for Nursing School.

Alana Hamilton was petite, barely five feet tall, with an array of freckles across the bridge of her nose and startling green eyes. She enjoyed her half hour runs at the end of the swim lessons.

When she ran through the park the swish of her Nike's barely made a sound. But he could hear her coming and so he waited.

He watched her run every afternoon for the

past week. Usually he just watched from the make shift campsite beneath the brooding evergreens but today was different, today he would follow her. Maybe touch the slivers of gold in her ponytail. Just touch. Nothing else, just touch.

Carl had been living in the park for a little over six months. His shelter was at the edge of the park close to the lake. It was an isolated area seldom used except for the occasional runner and of course the girl with the golden hair.

Before finding the park he'd been staying under the bridge downtown, but the crack smokers drove him away, pelted rocks at him till he finally decided to move. Nobody bothered him in the park, course no one knew he was there. A few times a week a couple of park attendants drove along the path but they never left their pickup truck and Carl had camouflaged his camp site well, taking care not to be seen. He seldom ate and the little food he needed he found in the dumpster behind the park cafe.

Usually Carl roamed the park late at night and slept in his burrow during daylight hours, but lately things had been changing. The voices were becoming more insistent, demanding almost. Telling him he had to prepare for the end. Find a family, prepare for the end.

ALANA SLOWED HER PACE

Alana slowed her pace, she could feel the sharp poke of a rock under the flap of her sneaker, up ahead she saw a bench, and she headed for it, flopped down and caught her breath. The wood was quiet, peaceful, but there was an uneasy feeling between her shoulder blades.

She looked around but could see nothing, still she felt as if someone were watching her. Foolishness, she scolded herself. It was just all the stress she'd been under this past month, always constant money problems and Grams health deteriorating rapidly and Kevin finally breaking up with her.

She should have called an end to their relationship months ago but didn't have the energy for it. Kevin wanted her to pack up and move to Texas after her dad died, but she couldn't do it, there was nobody to care for her grandmother. No one else to do the job, but Kevin couldn't understand her need to make sure her Gram was okay.

He finally gave her an ultimatum, go with him to Texas or he was going alone. He left last Tuesday by Friday she had been offered the instructor job at the aquatic center. Thank God for her job, perhaps now her life could get back on track.

Alana finished her run but she couldn't help

but feel someone watching her, she knew it was

a silly thought, but still the feeling persisted.

CARL

Carl watched as the golden girl left the park. He had missed his chance, but she would be back tomorrow, he knew this, the same way he knew many things. He gathered his army jacket around him and made his way deeper into the woods. He needed money for a bottle of Old Port. He had seven dollars a bottle of Old Port was almost twice that. He would need to venture towards were the lunch people sat. He could usually pick up enough cans and bottle to get his drink. It was risky though. Going where people sat exposed him, but he had a thirst that drove him on.

Sometimes along with the voices, Carl had flashes of memory of a time when he held a job as a correction officer. He once had a child and a wife. When he remembered the child the thirst and the need for the bottle of Old Port increased. His daughters name was Julie, but he didn't like to remember her. Mostly he didn't like to remember how he had killed them.

Carl trudged towards the picnic park, pulling his cap low across his eyes. He avoided the area where the banker sat. At least Carl thought he was a banker. The guy had the look of a banker or maybe an accountant, fancy three-piece suit, often carried a briefcase and an overcoat. Carl didn't like the guy. The guy came to the park once in awhile to feed the ducks. More than once Carl had seen the guy lure a duck in with food and then kick at it with the toe of his fancy dress shoe.

But maybe Carl was wrong maybe he just imagined what he saw, like the doctor in the emergency room told him. The Doc said his visions and his voices were just a part of his fucked up head and the constant drinking. Could be, didn't matter much to Carl one way or another. He had to get to the liquor store before it closed, that's all that mattered, that and maybe finding a woman before the end days. He shook his head and ran a trembling hand over his salt and pepper beard. Maybe he was nuts. He wasn't sure, maybe there was no such thing as the coming of the end days.

GRAM

Alana was hoping for a quick shower, a few minutes on her Facebook page to catch up with friends and maybe a chocolate latte when she saw the blinking lights of an ambulance parked out front of the town house she shared with her Gram. Her mouth got dry and her hands began to shake. She stepped up her pace, fearful of what she might find. She could see two paramedics coming down the step, one was munching on a big molasses cookie, surely they wouldn't be laughing if something terrible had happened.

Alana could barely voice the words, "is

everything okay in there?"

"And you are?" the taller once asked.

"Alana Hamilton, I live here with my Gram, is she okay?"

"Right as rain, but you might want to remind her, not to call 911, just to make sure everything is working. Dispatch took the call, she told them she felt a little dizzy and had an ache in her chest and then when we got here, she said she felt okay and gave us molasses cookies, vitals are fine, colour is good. I wouldn't exactly call it a prank call. But it sure is skating thin ice."

"I'll talk to her, not that it will do any good."

The tall paramedic patted Alana on the head,

people were always patting Alana on the head, sometimes she wished she were six foot four. "They wont charge her for this call, but it could get her in trouble," and he added, "Sometime she might really need us."

Alana wasn't looking forward to her conversation with her Gram life was becoming harder for Gram with each passing day. First Alana's dad passed away, and now Grams health was becoming progressively worse, her hearing was bad, she had developed cataracts and her diabetes was all over the place. But Alana was determined to finally have it out with her.

Alana marched up the steps determined to have it out with her grandmother, but when she opened the door she could see her grandmother sitting at the kitchen table her head in her hands, tears falling down her cheeks.

"Oh Gram, what is the matter?"

Her grandmother took a tissue out of her calico apron and dabbed at her eyes." I miss your grandfather so very much."

"I know you do Gram, I know you do."

"Those boys who came here to help me reminded me of him a little, in their uniforms you know. Your grandfather was a soldier when we first met."

Alana had never known her Grandfather, he died when Alana was still a baby. "And now with your father Gerald gone, it seems like all the men are dead. What are we going to do Alana, what are we going to do?"

Alana moved to stand behind her grandmother and began to give the elderly woman a neck massage. "We are going to pick ourselves up and put one foot in front of the other and go on Gram, you know you always told me that."

Alana bent down and kissed her grandmothers cheek, "and you dear lady are not going to call the paramedics unless you really, really need them, right."

The old woman wiped her nose with her soggy tissue, "you're right my dear, I know you are."

JEROME

Jerome Westchester the Third, tossed his Starbucks cup in the bushes and wiped the muffin crumbs from his fingers. He was in no hurry to get back to the office. Although if he strayed too long his significant other Sandra Wilcox might pout, but so what, the only thing significant about Sandra was that her daddy owned the company and was loaded.

Sandra was a dumpling and about as exciting as a rotten mushroom on a slice of pizza. She really did disgust him, but the way Jerome figured it, he only had to wait another few months before Sandra could disappear forever off the side of the sailboat and he, as dutiful son-in-law could comfort dear old dad.

It never ceased to amaze Jerome just how gullible people could be. Of course Jerome was good, he'd never been caught at anything that would cast a shadow on his character, his manners were impeccable, he was handsome and one of the sharpest dressers in the city. Everyone liked Jerome, everyone except perhaps that silly old drunk that Jerome sometimes saw slinking around the park. The drunk seemed to go out of his way to avoid Jerome, even when Jerome had held out a twenty dollar bill towards him one day. Jerome was sure the louse infested character would come forward and get the money, but he never did.

Jerome knew he probably shouldn't be hunting in the city where he lived, but it added to the excitement, and Jerome could feel the need to own a chickadee in his hand rising within him. It had been almost a year since the little redhead down in Toledo, just thinking about the way she squirmed when he held her throat in his hands was getting him hard.

He wondered what it would be like to grab the petite blond he saw leave the park, how surprised she would be when he wrapped his hands over her mouth, he would whisper in her ear, tell her every thing would be fine if she would just lie still while he fucked her.

She would comply. They always did. Thinking it would be easier to live with rape than to die, but they always died. Five was his current score, and Jerome knew he was destined to add more to his list. The question was, did he dare to hunt this close to home.

The more he thought about it, the more he realized it was exactly what he wanted to do. He could feel his erection pushing against his expensive trousers. Maybe he would go back to his office, close his door and push Sandra facedown against his desk, he would push her hard from behind, she would love it, even think he was overcome with passion for her, the silly bitch.

CARL'S BOTTLE

Carl's bottle of Old Port was past the half way mark before he had managed to stop thinking about his daughter Julie. The way her hair hung down her back almost to her waist, how she skipped along the pathways, singing in a childish voice. She loved the squirrels and ducks and they would bring breadcrumbs to feed them. She would hold his hand and swing it high in the sky asking him if he could catch the treetops for her.

Tears slid down Carl's cheeks running into his matted beard. Five years since he had gotten them killed and still the memory was as crystal clear as the trembling of his hands.

Saturday, July 3, five years ago at a little past supper time, he kissed Julie and Jessy good bye, gave them both a quick hug and headed in for his night shift at the correction centre. He seldom worked nights but a buddy was getting married in a few days and had asked Carl to switch so the buddy could attend his own bachelor party. Carl had agreed, he figured there would come a time when he would appreciate the favour. Maybe even next month when he would take the family and drive over to the coast. Julie had been asking him for ages to go see the ocean and Jessy would appreciate the break.

Carl fobbed himself through the set of steel doors and stood in the sally port while the brother manning master control open the next set of steel doors. There would only be the four of them manning the station during night shifts, him, Leroy, Sammy and Jason, they were all a good bunch and it would be an easy night.

"Heh Cal, Barry says to say thank you for switching, says he really appreciates it and he owes you one."

Carl walked through the metal detector and

then behind the Plexiglas office doors. He was in a virtual Plexiglas bubble, surrounded on all sides and able to see clearly down long hallways. There were a series of monitors arrayed across the desks. A board covered with keys, and a set of walkie talkies, belts, and PALS numbered in sequence, already being recorded by Sammy and his shift partner Leroy.

"All quiet on the home front tonight?" he asked of the two other officers already seated at the cameras.

"Easy peasy night we are going to have tonight bro." Said Jason Tremblay, he was the clown of the unit, but no-one ever gave him any sass. He was six foot four and three hundred pounds of rock hard muscle. But Jason rarely had to use his bulk, he had an easy going way of relaxing the inmates and settling an issue before it escalated. Carl envied him his relaxed manner with the inmates. It was a skill he hadn't yet mastered.

"Say, Carl how did the debrief go with the Captain last week. I heard you and Lena had a bit of trouble with a take down in C block."

"Yeah, it was tough" Carl didn't want to blame the fracas on Lena, even though the Captain had intimated as much.

Jason hung up the last of the change of shift keys on the count board. "Keys accounted for" he stated to the rest of the night shift crew. "Working with that wench is tricky for everyone, if there is anyone in the whole place that can stir up trouble, it's Lena, I'm surprised she hasn't gotten someone killed."

Sammy stopped his recording of the PALS long enough to say, "heard you had to press your PAL and call a code from other units."

Carl recalled the relief he'd felt when the riot squad showed up with shields and batons. "Yep, it sure was touch and go for a bit there. I thought for sure the whole place was gonna erupt. I'm not even sure how it got started in the first place. I think big Al Harnish accused Corker of cheating at poker and then someone called someone the N word and next thing you know a fight broke out.

Lena and I arrived after Blake threw a punch

at Charlie and big Al had Corker on the floor in a head lock and Blake was bloodied with a shiv. Never did find out who stabbed him, but Lena blamed Giovanni and cracked him on the head with her walkie talkie and for some reason Giovanni thought it was me who slugged him, threatened to cut my fucking balls off and feed em to the fish. Anyway it settled down once the code guys arrived."

Jason adjusted one of the monitors so he could get a better view of a group of inmates seated around the television set. "You know Cal I'd keep my eye on my truck tires if I were you. I wouldn't trust Giovanni an inch. But you won't have to worry about it I guess, at least for a year or two, till he shows back up again, heard they released him this morning. Good thing too, I heard he still had a hate on for you."

Carl relaxed just a little, he was glad Giovanni was off the range. He didn't need the friction. He gathered the board and told Sammy he would go with him for the live body checks. He and Sammy made half hour checks and the night was uneventful until a little after 0315 when Captain Larkin, a police detective Carl didn't know, the Chaplain, Father Mike, and a CW from B block, who Carl recognized from the cafeteria, showed up.

It didn't make sense to have these guys coming making rounds in the middle of the night. The range had been quiet, as far as Carl could tell all the inmates were locked in and asleep. Carl couldn't figure out what would be so urgent it couldn't wait until morning but he opened the steel doors to the Sally port to let the men into the station.

Carl wasn't Catholic, but he and Father Mike often played a round of pick up basketball Saturday mornings, he liked the guy, he was a big friendly Irishman, but he looked grim, and Captain Larkin who Carl respected greatly seemed ill at ease.

The Captain spoke first, "Carl, get your things together, Joey here from B block will finish your shift for you. You need to come with me and Detective Angelo."

Carl could feel a churning deep in his gut, "What's up Cap?"

"Just come with me Carl."

Father Michael reached out and touched Carl on the arm, Carl didn't think he had ever seen more sorrow on a man's face. "It's Jessy and Julie, Carl, there's been an incident involving Giovanni Alusso."

"Giovanni Alusso, what the fuck's Giovanni got to do with Jessy and Julie, don't dick with me Mike, you're talking about my wife and my baby, my family. They don't know Giovanni, shit I don't know Giovanni."

"They're all dead Carl," and that is the last thing Carl heard that night. Later he learned Giovanni had strapped himself with home made explosives marched up to Carl's door and preceded to blow up himself, Carl's wife, and

Carl's seven year old daughter Julie. In a less than ten seconds every reason Carl ever had for living was gone. Carl started drinking and hadn't seen a sober day in over five years. He functioned sort of, but not really. Nothing mattered to him anymore, not his hygiene or his health, nothing.

ALANA & SANDRA

Alana finished drying her hair, when Jake Wilcox's Aunt Sandra poked her head in Alana's office door. "I just wanted to tell you how pleased I am with the progress Jake is making. All he ever says is Miss Hamilton this and Miss Hamilton that, I think he has a crush on you Alana."

Alana smiled, "He is coming along, that is for sure, he tells me he has to learn to swim because you are getting married in a month and he wants to be able to swim when you all go to Aruba for the ceremonies."

"I have never seen him so happy, you certainly do have a way with young children. It seems like a lot of people have difficulty relating to downs syndrome kids but if Jake is any indication, you've found a way to work with these kids that is astounding, and I really did want to thank you."

"It is my pleasure, Miss Wilcox, Jake is a very loving child and determined to please you." Alana didn't want to bring up the subject but it did seem important. "He keeps talking about not wanting to swim for that tight wadded booger rat, and I am not sure who he is referring to."

Sandra gave a nervous laugh. "Jake is my only

nephew, and I adore him, I always have, but for the life of me I cannot figure out why he dislikes my finance so much."

Sandra held out her hand and showed Alana an exquisite solitaire diamond. "We've only known each other three months, and been engaged for two. I admit it has been sort of a whirlwind courtship and maybe that is it. Or maybe it is Jakes age, he is thirteen and, well I guess he has never seen me paying much attention to any males other than him. I do so wish he would warm up to Jerome though."

"Oh, maybe it will just take some time. Kids with Jake's challenges either love you to pieces or don't like you at all. It might be he just needs a little more time."

"Perhaps Alana you are right, maybe you would be so kind as to help me with Jake just a little. It would mean so much to me. He obviously adores you and perhaps, well I was wondering, we are having a small get together Sunday afternoon and well, I was wondering if perhaps you might attend. Jerome will be there of course and, maybe if Jake sees you chatting with Jerome he will start to warm up to him. Do you think you could possibly attend?"

Alana wasn't so sure she really wanted to spend an afternoon with people she barely knew, but the Wilcox family was very prominent in the city, and Mr. Samuel Wilcox had been one of the people who had hired her for the job and she really did want to make a good impression and she was particularly fond of Jake. "I would be delighted,", she said, who knows maybe it would ease his relations with Miss Wilcox fiancé and that would be a bonus for Jake.

"Oh, thank you so very much, I will send the chauffeur around for you at two, if that is all right?"

"Two will be fine, would it be okay if I brought my grandmother, I don't like to leave her alone on the weekends if I can help it."

"No of course not, by all means bring her along, like I say it will just be a casual Sunday get together. I had heard you were the caretaker for your grandmother. In fact quite frankly Alana being a caretaker for your grandmother was one of the reasons the board hired you, if I recall correctly."

"Thank you Miss Wilcox, I will be looking forward to the Sunday gathering and I am sure Gram will be delighted."

"Call me Sandi, everyone does. See you on Sunday then."

THE END

TO BE CONTINUED...

ABOUT THE AUTHOR

Carolyn Ann Vaughan writes stories with nursing characters. Her first novel, *Secret Diaries of a Nurse: and other short stories,* is a collection of stories, some complete and two listed as *to be continued*, one a thriller *The Jagged Edge* and the other a romance called *Lydia's folly* with nursing characters.

Carolyn Ann Vaughan was born in Lunenburg County, Nova Scotia, Canada, within spitting distance of Captain Kidd's famous Oak Island.

She was educated in Ontario, and at the age of thirty, when her son Michael and her daughters Heather and Melissa were four, six and eight she attended Mac School of Nursing. She graduated from nursing school with the second highest mark in the province of Ontario.

She worked as a Registered Nurse for many years, in three provinces, one American state, and a Native Reservation. She has three adult children, a son and two daughters and two grandsons (Morgan and Devun) as well as an extended family, step daughter Sarah, daughter in law Jennifer, and step son Michael and step grandson Jordan.

Along with passion for her writing she enjoys gardening quilting, and playing guitar on her YouTube channel.

She currently lives in Dartmouth Nova Scotia with her soul mate David (also an RN) and three goldfish.

Carolyn Ann Vaughan RN